D1565250

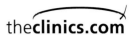

NURSING CLINICS OF NORTH AMERICA

Dermatologic Nursing

GUEST EDITOR
Heather Jones, RN, BSN

CONSULTING EDITOR
Suzanne S. Prevost, PhD, RN

September 2007 • Volume 42 • Number 3

SAUNDERS

An Imprint of Elsevier, Inc.
PHILADELPHIA   LONDON   TORONTO   MONTREAL   SYDNEY   TOKYO

W.B. SAUNDERS COMPANY
A Division of Elsevier Inc.

1600 John F. Kennedy Blvd., Suite 1800, Philadelphia, PA 19103-2899

http://www.theclinics.com

NURSING CLINICS OF NORTH AMERICA   Volume 42, Number 3
September 2007   ISSN 0029-6465
Editor: Ali Gavenda   ISBN-13: 978-1-4160-5096-4
    ISBN-10: 1-4160-5096-5

The ideas and opinions expressed in *Nursing Clinics of North America* do not necessarily reflect those of the Publisher. The Publisher does not assume any responsibility for any injury and/or damage to persons or property arising out of or related to any use of the material contained in this periodical. The reader is advised to check the appropriate medical literature and the product information currently provided by the manufacturer of each drug to be administered to verify the dosage, the method and duration of administration, or contraindications. It is the responsibility of the treating physician or other health care professional, relying on independent experience and knowledge of the patient, to determine drug dosages and the best treatment for the patient. Mention of any product in this issue should not be construed as endorsement by the contributors, editors, or the Publisher of the product or manufacturers' claims.

Nursing Clinics of North America (ISSN 0029-6465) is published quarterly by Elsevier Inc., 360 Park Avenue South, New York, NY 10010-1710. Months of issue are March, June, September, and December. Business and Editorial Offices: 1600 John F. Kennedy Blvd., Suite 1800, Philadelphia, PA 19103-2899. Customer Service Office: 6277 Sea Harbor Drive, Orlando, FL 32887-4800. Periodicals postage paid at New York, NY and additional mailing offices. Subscription price per year is, $116.00 (US individuals), $216.00 (US institutions), $187.00 (international individuals), $259.00 (international institutions), $160.00 (Canadian individuals), $259.00 (Canadian institutions), $61.00 (US students), and $94.00 (international students). To receive student/resident rate, orders must be accompanied by name of affiliated institution, date of term, and the signature of program/residency coordinator on institution letterhead. Orders will be billed at individual rate until proof of status is received. Foreign air speed delivery is included in all *Clinics* subscription prices. All prices are subject to change without notice. **POSTMASTER:** Send address changes to *Nursing Clinics*, Elsevier Periodicals Customer Service, 6277 Sea Harbor Drive, Orlando, FL 32887-4800. **Customer Service: 1-800-654-2452 (US). From outside of the US, call 1-407-345-4000.**

Nursing Clinics of North America is covered in *EMBASE/Excerpta Medica, Index Medicus, Social Sciences Citation Index, Current Contents, ASCA, Cumulative Index to Nursing, RNdex Top 100*, and *Allied Health Literature and International Nursing Index (INI)*.

Printed in the United States of America.

CONSULTING EDITOR

SUZANNE S. PREVOST, PhD, RN, Nursing Professor and National HealthCare Chair of Excellence, Middle Tennessee State University, School of Nursing, Murfreesboro, Tennessee

GUEST EDITOR

HEATHER JONES, RN, BSN, Dermatologic and Cutaneous Laser Surgery, Department of Dermatology, Oregon Health & Science University, Portland, Oregon

CONTRIBUTORS

LAKSHI M. ALDREDGE, RN, MSN, ANP, Dermatology Service, Portland VA Medical Center, Portland, Oregon

PAULA E. BERMANN, MSN, RN, APRN, BC, DNC, Dermatology Clinical Nurse Specialist/Nurse Practitioner, Savannah, Georgia

PATRICIA GILLEAUDEAU, RN, MSN, FNP, Research Nurse Practitioner, The Rockefeller University, Laboratory of Investigative Dermatology, New York, New York

CLAIR HOLLISTER, LVN, Department of Dermatology, University of California, San Diego, La Jolla, California

HEATHER JONES, RN, BSN, Dermatologic and Cutaneous Laser Surgery, Department of Dermatology, Oregon Health & Science University, Portland, Oregon

VINCENT W. LI, MD, Institute for Advanced Studies, The Angiogenesis Foundation, Cambridge; and The Angiogenesis Clinic, Department of Dermatology, Brigham and Women's Hospital, Boston, Massachusetts

SUE A. McCANN, MSN, RN, DNC, Advanced Practice Nurse, Photopheresis Nurse Coordinator, CTCL Research Coordinator, Department of Dermatology; and Department of Nursing, University of Pittsburgh Medical Center, Pittsburgh, Pennsylvania

LESLIE M. PLAUNTZ, RN, BA, DNC, Plastic Surgery Clinical Nurse Specialist, Division of Plastic Surgery, Sunnybrook Health Science Centres, Toronto, Ontario, Canada

MARY SULLIVAN-WHALEN, RN, MSN, FNP, Research Nurse Practitioner, The Rockefeller University, Laboratory of Investigative Dermatology, New York, New York

SUSAN TOFTE, RN, MS, FNP-C, Assistant Professor, Department of Dermatology, Oregon Health & Science University, Portland, Oregon

CONTENTS

Nurses play an important role in the preassessment of surgical patients. With the rise in free-standing surgical clinics and the move of many surgical procedures to office-based surgical clinics, quality patient care could be compromised. Preassessment of surgical patients in office-based and hospital clinics ensures quality patient care from the moment patients enter the office to when they are discharged from care. The process of preoperative evaluation is essential in assessing the medical condition of patients, evaluating their overall health status, determining risk factors, and educating them. Surgical preassessment benefits patients, physicians, and nurses by not only improving surgical outcomes and patient satisfaction but also ensuring patient safety. Nurses employed in office-based surgical suites require specialized knowledge and clinical skills to offer continued, well-informed care to their patients.

The role of sentinel lymph node biopsy (SLNB) as a prognostic indicator in melanoma patients has been controversial in the fields of surgical oncology and dermatology for decades. This minimally invasive surgical technique was introduced in 1990 for diagnosing melanoma lymphatic metastases and has been deemed the standard of surgical care of cutaneous malignant melanoma by the World Health Organization and the Sunbelt Melanoma Clinical Trial. Its usefulness as a prognostic indicator of metastases led to expanded applications for breast, colon, gastric, esophageal, head and neck, thyroid, and lung cancers. This article first provides an overview of cutaneous melanoma and staging methods and treatment modalities. A brief study of the lymphatic system and the SLNB procedure are reviewed, followed by a discussion of its usefulness in patients who have melanoma, including risks and benefits. This article also discusses nursing considerations for patients undergoing the procedure, and patient education tips. Lastly, future indications for SLNB and new prognostic indicators for melanoma are discussed.

Nurses have become an essential part of patient care in laser therapy. In dermatology, the potential for helping patients achieve excellent results for individual skin needs is exponential when combined with appropriate technology, evidence-based care, and a competent, conscientious nurse. This article explains how a laser functions, outlines the use of lasers in treating particular dermatologic conditions, provides guidelines for posttreatment care, and discusses the nurse's role in providing laser treatment.

Atopic dermatitis (AD) is a chronic inflammatory skin disease characterized by intense pruritus and frequent relapsing courses. It occurs mostly in patients who have a personal or family history of other atopic conditions, such as asthma or allergic rhinitis. The prevalence of AD is high, particularly in children, with rapidly increasing numbers in the past few decades. The chronicity of this disease, along with its relapsing nature, presents treatment and management challenges for clinicians and frustration for patients and their families.

Cutaneous T-cell lymphoma (CTCL) is an uncommon and complex malignancy of the immune system with a wide range of clinical presentations primarily involving the skin. An extensive menu of skin-directed and/or systemic treatment options exists. Best practices in management involve multidisciplinary collaboration. Nursing care for patients who have CTCL is a critical component in the successful management of the disease and requires special attention to the patient's physical, emotional, and spiritual needs.

Nurses can make a significant impact by being accessible, offering emotional support, demonstrating advocacy, and providing ongoing education for the patient and family.

FORTHCOMING ISSUES

RECENT ISSUES

ELSEVIER
SAUNDERS

Nurs Clin N Am 42 (2007) ix–x

NURSING
CLINICS
OF NORTH AMERICA

Preface

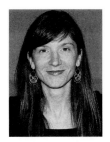

Heather Jones, RN, BSN
Guest Editor

Dermatology is an exciting and rapidly changing specialty. The breadth of knowledge can be overwhelming, yet incredibly intriguing. The skin is the most observable part of the human body. Considering this, one is commonly aware of changes in their skin. In turn, most nurses, regardless of specialty, will encounter patients seeking care for their dermatology needs.

My intentions with this issue of the *Nursing Clinics of North America* are threefold. I hope to reach an audience of nurses who have yet to consider how fundamental skin disease knowledge can be in their professional role, increasing their desire to gain more dermatology knowledge. Next, I hope to provide new information for dermatology nurse colleagues, who may find new, fascinating information that ignites their curiosity to broaden their dermatology knowledge bases. Finally, I hope to reach those new to nursing. I'd like to invite them to explore an area of medicine within which they may have never envisioned themselves.

Throughout these pages, you will learn from expert nurses in dermatology. These leading nurses will share their knowledge and experiences in such topics as nurse-administered laser, cutaneous T cell lymphoma, wound healing and angiogenesis, preoperative wound care, aging skin, and more. These authors provide the reader with an exceptional opportunity to see the many aspects of dermatology, while sharing with them years of dermatology experience, evidence-based information, and personal, caring perspectives.

I would like to extend a sincere thank you to all of the contributors who have lent their time and knowledge to this book. These are individuals who

0029-6465/07/$ - see front matter © 2007 Elsevier Inc. All rights reserved.
doi:10.1016/j.cnur.2007.07.003
nursing.theclinics.com

have been willing to share their expertise not only in direct patient care, but through professional organizations, peer education, and publication. Their willingness to go beyond their role as caregiver, to the role of educator, ensures a future of enhanced patient outcomes. Their hard work and dedication to teaching is noble and is a credit to themselves, their patients, and all nurses.

Heather Jones, RN, BSN
Dermatologic and Cutaneous Laser Surgery
Department of Dermatology
Oregon Health & Science University
3303 SW Bond Avenue
Portland, OR 97229, USA

E-mail address: joneshea@ohsu.edu

NURSING
CLINICS
OF NORTH AMERICA

ELSEVIER
SAUNDERS

Nurs Clin N Am 42 (2007) 361–377

Preoperative Assessment
of the Surgical Patient

Leslie M. Plauntz, RN, BA, DNC

Division of Plastic Surgery, Sunnybrook Health Science Centres,
14 Rappert Avenue, Toronto, Ontario, M4P 2V2, Canada

Nurses play an important role in the preassessment of surgical patients. More than one third of the members of the Dermatology Nurses Association (DNA) work in office-based practices [1]. Many of these offices perform dermatologic procedures, such as biopsies and Mohs micrographic surgery, and a growing number of cosmetic surgeries. Office-based practices have multiplied because of key benefits, such as reduced patient cost, ease of scheduling, reduced incidence of hospital-acquired infections, and overall convenience to patients and surgeons. Although office-based surgery is a growing trend in surgical services offered to many patients, it has risks [2]. Office-based procedures are associated with an estimated 10-fold increase in risk for serious injury or death compared with procedures performed in ambulatory surgical facilities [3]. Increases in surgical risks have been attributed to insufficient time spent performing preoperative assessment, providing preoperative teaching, and assessing postoperative complications. Regardless of cost-containment and added convenience to patients and surgeons, patient safety must always take precedence [4]. With the continued rise in office-based surgery, the office nurse holds a key position in assessing patient health status before surgery, planning the perioperative experience, and monitoring, instructing, and evaluating surgical patients through all stages of surgery.

Purpose

This article addresses the importance of preassessment of surgical patients, discusses how the growth of outpatient surgery has impacted office-based practices, and provides recommendations for outpatient office-based surgical clinics to ensure quality patient care, especially in the preoperative phase of surgery.

E-mail address: leslie.plauntz@sunnybrook.ca

The preoperative phase describes nursing care from the time surgical intervention is decided until patients are transferred to the surgical suite. The process of preoperative evaluation is essential in assessing the medical condition of patients, evaluating their overall health status, determining risk factors, and educating patients while giving them time to discuss the procedure in detail. In return, the patient gains a realistic understanding of the proposed surgery and realizes the possible complications that could occur during the perioperative period [5]. The risks versus benefits of surgery and surgical limitations must be clearly outlined for patients during the preoperative interview. Patients who are determined to be of a high surgical risk have a higher propensity for perioperative and postoperative mortality and morbidity [6]. Office staff, nurses, and physicians all play a large role in the preoperative phase, because quality patient care begins when patients enter the office and continues until they are discharged.

Background

Medical technology and health care delivery have changed dramatically during the past 15 years. The largest shift has been the relocation of surgical offices, which has resulted in patients undergoing more surgical procedures in ambulatory settings and freestanding surgical centers [7,8]. The movement of many surgical procedures from the hospital to office-based surgical centers has contributed to the increase in office-based, ambulatory same-day, and outpatient surgery. In 1996, outpatient surgery accounted for 31.5 million procedures [9]. The American Society for Dermatologic Surgery surveyed their members in 2002 and found that dermatologists performed 3.9 million procedures in 2002, with skin cancer surgery being the most common, at 1.4 million [10]. This study also suggested that dermatologists perform a broad range of dermatology surgery within their offices, beyond simple excisions of skin cancer. Examples of these surgeries include liposuction, hair transplants, and skin resurfacing [11]. Experts believe that the trend for increased elective procedures in office-based and outpatient settings will continue.

Growth of cosmetic procedures and the effect on office-based procedures

Increased cosmetic procedures has been a major contributor to the shift from hospital inpatient settings to ambulatory settings and freestanding centers. In 2004, surgical cosmetic procedures such as liposuction and facelifts, and nonsurgical cosmetic procedures such as Botox (Allergan Inc., Irvine, CA) and collagen increased in the United States to 11.9 million. The growth of cosmetic procedures in 2004 represents a 44% increase over 2003. The strengthening economy, aging of the baby boomers, and people becoming more willing to invest in ways to make them feel good about their appearance all contribute to the rise in office-based procedures [12]. The top five surgical cosmetic procedures contributing to the growth in plastic surgery in 2005 were liposuction, breast augmentation, blepharoplasty (eyelid surgery), abdominoplasty (tummy tuck), and breast lift. The top five nonsurgical cosmetic procedures in 2005 were Botox injections, laser hair removal, hyaluronic acid, microdermabrasion, and chemical peels. Most surgical and nonsurgical cosmetic procedures (76%) were performed either in an office facility or a freestanding surgical clinic [10]. Although many nonsurgical procedures are considered simple and may not require extensive preassessment, all surgical procedures require a health preassessment to properly evaluate patient safety for undergoing office-based surgery procedures.

Surgical risk of office-based practices

With the rise in cosmetic procedures and office-based surgery, more patients return home the same day of surgery rather than stay overnight in hospitals. Early discharge of patients can result in an increased risk to patient safety. At least 44,000 Americans are reported to die annually from preventable medical errors. Furthermore, medical mistakes are the leading cause of death in the United States, costing between $54.6 billion and $79 billion, or 6% of total annual national health care expenditures [3]. Surprisingly, most studies show that surgical complications in outpatient procedures relate to anesthesia, general or laparoscopic surgery, or orthopedic and head and neck procedures, not dermatology skin surgery [13]. Bitar and colleagues [13] evaluated the safety and efficacy of 3615 consecutive patients undergoing office-based surgery under monitored anesthesia care/sedation in a single office between May 1995 and May 2000. This study concluded that office-based surgery can be safe for the patient if proper precautions are taken, including appropriate accreditation, safe anesthesia protocols, presence of educated well-informed staff, and proper patient selection.

Rise in office-based surgery and its effect on nursing

Shortage of experienced nurses

The increase in office-based practices has challenged the skill competencies and educational requirements of nurses in ambulatory settings. Contributing to problems in office-based practices is the shortage of trained experienced nurses available to staff surgical suites. The shortage of well-trained nurses is related to decreased enrollment in baccalaureate nursing programs and early retirement. The American Association of Colleges of Nursing (2003) reports that since 1995, enrollment in nursing programs has declined 17%. Also, calculations show that approximately half of the registered nurse workforce will reach retirement age in the next 15 years [14]. In a recent survey conducted by the American Nurses Association, the average age of retirement was reported to be as young as 45.2 years

[15]. Further aggravating the situation is the fact that new registered nurses are leaving the workforce at far faster rates than their predecessors [16]. These facts all contribute to a workforce of uneducated, underskilled nurses. The quality of patient care could be compromised because of deficiencies in knowledge, skills, judgment, and ability to interpret health findings by staff caring for patients, in both the hospital setting and office-based practices.

Education of office staff

Staff must be educated in preassessment protocols and the health requirements that all patients must meet before surgery. Preassessment ensures better understanding and knowledge of patients' health history and how it may affect their health status during and after surgery. This health history is essential, because it guides the focus the physical examination, identifies appropriate nursing procedures, and helps nurses plan patient and family care before surgery and postoperatively. Patient preassessment and education remain major factors in ensuring patient safety in office-based settings, and are areas in which nurses can play a large role.

The Association of Operating Room Nurses states that nursing practice in the ambulatory surgical setting should recognize the significance and importance of skilled nurses who are clinically and professionally competent to provide skilled nursing care to their patients. Preoperative nursing assessments and patient education are vital elements in providing quality care to patients undergoing all types of surgical procedures [17]. Therefore, a complete patient assessment, including a thorough review of the medical record, past medical illnesses, or prior surgical procedures, is essential in establishing patients' baseline physical and psychological parameters before they undergo surgery. Clinical outcomes in office-based surgical suites can be improved with a thorough and complete premedical assessment of all patients. The clinical aspects of patient safety also require that physicians evaluate whether the procedures and patients are appropriate for the office setting. Physicians and office staff who give the healing touch of quality care must always have patient safety as the foremost priority [3].

The literature on ambulatory care management offers information and suggests several factors that may increase risks in office-based practices:

- Tendency to operate on patients who do not meet safety criteria for outpatient operations (eg, many complex conditions, too complex of an operation)
- Lack of appropriate safety measures and protocols, policies, and procedures (eg, credentialing, privileging) to ensure the training and experience of staff performing surgery or to manage sedation and anesthesia
- Greater variation in how well equipment is maintained (eg, monitoring devices)
- Few standards in the education, training, and experience of personnel using equipment and caring for patients [2,18]

Every surgical office should have standards that address patient safety, preassessment protocols, staff training, and accreditation of the surgical suite. Office-based staff need time to access critical medical history of patients before any surgery is performed. The American Association of Nurse Anesthetists (AANA) advocate high-quality appropriate standards of care for all patients in all settings, including the office-based practice setting. The AANA has outlined standards regarding practitioner qualifications, training, equipment, facilities, and policies that ensure patient safety [18]. The AANA advocates that a thorough and complete preanesthesia assessment be performed for all patients, including a review of physical status, previous anesthetic history, allergies, medical history, and physical examination. The AANA's Standards for Office-Based Anesthesia Practice is an excellent reference and model for office-based practices [19].

The nurse's role in preassessment of surgical patients

Recommendations for preoperative history and physical examination

The purpose of a health assessment is to collect data in an organized manner, analyze and synthesize the data, use the data to guide the physical assessment, perform nursing actions, and initiate a patient/family teaching and educational plan before surgery. The format for obtaining a health history is usually combined with the taking of a health history from either the patient, past medical records, referrals from other physicians, or other health care providers. The health history includes history of present illness, signs or symptoms of current or past illnesses, diagnostic tests, current health status, comorbid factors, and significant/associated family history.

The role of the nurse in a health assessment is to collect information that helps determine the patient's current health status. A detailed evaluation of a patient's health history allows physicians and nurses to be aware of any potential problems that could occur in the preoperative or postoperative phase of surgery. With this information, nurses can develop a plan of treatment, identify and minimize risk factors, and involve support systems if necessary [20]. In more complex surgeries such as invasive facial skin cancers, specialties such as general surgery, oncology, or plastic surgery may need to be consulted before surgery.

Some dermatologic procedures, such as cryosurgery, curettage, and punch biopsies, are uncomplicated and do not require extensive medical histories, whereas more complex dermatology procedures, such as hair transplants, flaps, and graphs, require a detailed evaluation of a patient's health history [5]. However, social history (tobacco or alcohol use), history of allergies, use of medications (prescribed, illicit, and over-the-counter), and previous anesthetic problems should be reviewed for every patient.

Patients in most ambulatory hospital settings are required to complete a Preoperative Patient Questionnaire. Included on this form are medications, allergies, medical history, surgical history, general health history, and details concerning any past significant illnesses. The patient can complete the form either independently or with the assistance of the nurse. Completion of the form allows for a complete and concise review of the patient's health history. After the form is completed, a health professional should review all areas of the health history with the patient.

In the Surgical Mohs unit at Women's College Hospital in Toronto, Ontario, all patients complete not only the preoperative questionnaire form but also spend time with the nurse before undergoing Mohs surgery. Time with the nurse allows patients to clarify medication use, review their medical history, and have the opportunity to ask questions about the surgery. Preoperative patient education helps patients understand the surgical experience, minimizes anxiety, and promotes full recovery from surgery and anesthesia. The perioperative nurse can assess the patient's knowledge base and use this information in developing a patient care plan that will ensure an uneventful perioperative course [21]. Patients must be well informed about all aspects of their surgery, including risks, benefits, what can be done, what cannot be done, and what are realistic expectations of the surgical outcome. The office nurse can play a large role in not only discussing the health history but also helping patients have reasonable expectations, especially with elective cosmetic procedures. Both nurses and physicians must be fully informed about all aspects of a patient's health history. Equally, patients must be fully informed about their surgery. Educating patients before surgery reduces anxiety and helps them have a more realistic understanding of possible surgical outcomes. Box 1 summarizes the elements involved in a preoperative basic health assessment.

Box 1. Preoperative basic health assessment

A complete preoperative basic health assessment includes
Medical history
Indication for surgical procedure
Allergies and reaction type to specific medication
Known medical problems
Surgical history
Current medications (prescription and nonprescription)

Focused review of health issues that relate to the planned anesthesia/procedure
Current known medical conditions
Cardiac status
Hematologic system
Infections
Pulmonary status

Personal or family history of bleeding problems
Anemia
Pregnancy
Past personal or family history of anesthesia problems
Smoking and alcohol history
Previous healing and scarring problems

Physical examination
Weight/height
Vital signs, blood pressure, pulse (rate and regularity),
    respiratory rate
Cardiac
Pulmonary
Other pertinent examinations

Possible tests
Hemoglobin if patient has history of anemia, if significant blood
    loss is anticipated
Potassium if patient is taking diuretics
Coagulation studies if patient has a history of recent bleeding or
    coagulation abnormalities
Chest radiograph if. patient has signs or symptoms of new
    or unstable cardiopulmonary disease
ECG if patient is older than 55 years or has a history of diabetes,
    hypertension, chest pain, smoking, peripheral vascular
    disease, or morbid obesity [22]

Psychological care
Minor dermatologic/oncologic patients
    Help reduce patient anxiety
Cosmetic dermatology patients
    Help patient have realistic expectations

Initial diagnostic assessment

Initial diagnostic assessment should include a review of past and current medical conditions, existing and past medical patient health history, and family health risks.

Medical conditions and current health history

Diabetes mellitus

Poorly controlled diabetics may cause adverse wound healing and increase chance of infection. Blood glucose levels and insulin doses should be monitored and controlled before surgery.

Hypertension

Patients who have elevated blood pressures may bleed profusely, especially in highly vascular areas such as the scalp. Adequate pain control in the perioperative phase is important to prevent hypertension, which could lead to bleeding and hematoma formation and compromise healing.

Cardiovascular disease

Epinephrine use in local anesthetics may have vasoconstrictive and cardiostimulatory effects. Patents who have valvular heart disease or prosthetic valves have a greater risk for developing endocarditis. History of valvular heart disease, mitral stenosis, rheumatic heart disease, or infective endocarditis should be noted. A course of prophylactic antibiotics may be indicated [5]. Recommendations for antibiotic prophylaxis change often; the American Heart Association guidelines for preventing bacterial endocarditis provide more information. Patients who have cardiac pacemakers or defibrillators should be identified. Because electrocautery may cause pacemaker interference, the patient's cardiologist should be consulted before surgery.

Organ transplants/artificial joints

Patients who have undergone organ transplantation or joint replacement may require prophylactic antibiotics, especially if transplant surgery was performed recently. Patients who have total joint replacements, are immunosuppressed, have rheumatoid arthritis, have systemic lupus, are type 1 insulin–dependent, have a history of previous prosthetic joint infections, or are malnourished should receive antibiotic prophylaxis before surgery [5].

Respiratory

Patients who have a preoperative history of chronic obstructive pulmonary disease, productive cough, cigarette smoking, obesity, and abnormal findings on both physical examination and chest radiograph are at an increased risk for adverse effects from general anesthesia. Consultation with an anesthetist is indicated before surgery, especially when patients will receive a general anesthetic.

Risk for bleeding

Abnormalities related to a past history of excessive bleeding should be screened. If suspected, a complete blood count, platelet count, prothrombin time, and an activated partial thromboplastin time should be obtained.

Seizure disorders/stroke

Past cerebrovascular accidents should always be noted. Because patients may have heart disease and be on an antiplatelet (aspirin) or anticoagulant (heparin, warfarin), nurses should determine whether these drugs can be safely discontinued before surgery.

Nutrition

Vitamin A, C, and K deficiencies impair normal wound healing.

Herpes simplex virus

A history of herpes simplex virus may require the use of an antiviral prophylaxis, such as acyclovir.

Cardiovascular system

Congestive heart failure, unstable angina, or recent myocardial infarct requires patients to undergo a cardiac workup before undergoing a surgical procedure. When patients have a history of heart disease and are receiving a general anesthetic, an anesthetist should be consulted before surgery.

Pregnancy

Nonemergent procedures should be postponed until postpartum. Lidocaine is safe in low doses, although excessive amounts can cause fetal central nervous system and cardiac depression. Acetaminophen (class B) is routinely used during pregnancy despite its ability to cross the placenta [5].

Psychiatric concerns

Current mental status should be assessed because this may affect a patient's understanding of surgery and willingness to cooperate with the treatment plan. Family members may need to be included in the preassessment workup and throughout the surgical process to support the patient.

Preoperative evaluation of allergies

Patients must always be questioned about all known allergies and drug sensitivities.

Local anesthetics

True allergic reactions are rare, and are usually caused by sensitivity to the paraben preservatives (methyl or propylparaben) [5]. Allergy testing is recommended before proceeding. Patients should always be questioned about allergies, even for minor procedures, to avoid anaphylactic reactions.

Adhesive/skin preparations/latex

Adhesive tape should be avoided when patients are sensitive. Latex allergies are a rising concern, with symptoms varying from localized urticaria to anaphylaxis. Incidence of allergy to natural rubber latex is increasing in health care workers, patients who undergo multiple surgeries, and atopic individuals. Vinyl or synthetic gloves should be available in the clinic.

Analgesics

Allergies to analgesics should always be noted and avoided.

Antibiotics

Allergies to antibiotics should also always be noted and avoided. Topical antibiotics, such as Polysporin ointment and Bactroban, can cause localized sensitization. Vaseline or petrolatum is a safe alternative to apply to wounds postoperatively.

Medications

Medications include all prescribed and over-the-counter medications. Aspirin and nonsteroidal anti-inflammatory inhibit platelet function. Nurses should always check with a pharmacist when they are unsure about ingredients in a medication and should question patients about the use of recreational drugs or alcohol; both should be discontinued before and after surgery to improve wound healing. Chronic use of alcohol can increase anesthetic requirements because reduced anesthetic metabolism and decreased liver function increase the risk for toxicity. Barbiturates may have a cardiac depressant effect and opioids, such as codeine phosphate and morphine HCI, may cause vasoconstriction, hypertension, and tachyarrhythmias mainly with general anesthetics. Vitamin supplements, such as vitamin E and alpha-omega vitamins, should be avoided preoperatively because they may increase the risk for bleeding.

Recommendations for blood thinners

Acetylsalicylic acid

Acetylsalicylic acid should be discontinued 5 to 7 days before surgery and restarted 5 to 7 days after surgery, although it can be restarted 1 day after surgery if medically necessary. Recommendations for acetylsalicylic acid may vary according to the medical reasons for use, and therefore the primary physician should always be consulted when patients are using prescribed medications.

Coumadin (warfarin sodium)

Coumadin inhibits platelet function. Patients are recommended to discontinue coumadin 3 days before surgery and restart it 1 day after surgery. For all blood thinners, one must always weigh risks over benefits and consult with the primary physician before discontinuing.

Box 2 lists the more common products containing aspirin and aspirin-like compounds. Patients should be advised to avoid the medications included on this list for 5 to 7 days before and after a surgical procedure. Patients should also avoid alcohol consumption and smoking for 2 weeks before surgery. This list is not complete; many other products may contain aspirin, aspirin-like compounds, or ibuprofen. Nurses should always check with

---

Box 2. Common medications containing aspirin, aspirin-like compounds, ibuprofen, naproxen, or naproxen sodium

Common nonprescription products containing aspirin or aspirin-like compounds
Alka-Seltzer Antacid/Pain Reliever
Bufferin Arthritis Strength Caplets
Effervescent Tablets
Bufferin Caplets/Tablets
Alka-Seltzer Plus Cold Medicine Tablets
Cama Arthritis Pain Reliever Tablets
Anacin Caplets/Tablets
Doan's Pills Caplets
Anacin Caplets/Tablets
Ecotrin Caplets/Tablets
Arthritis Pain Formula Tablets
Empirin Tablets
Arthritis Strength Bufferin Tablets
Excedrin Extra-Strength Caplets/Tablets
Bayer Aspirin Caplets/Tablets
P-A-C Analgesic/Tablets
Bayer Children's Chewable Tablets
Pepto-Bismol Liquid/Tablets
Bayer Plus Tablets
Sine-Off Tablets, Aspirin Formula
Maximum Bayer Caplets/Tablets
St. Joseph Adult Chewable Aspirin
8-Hour Bayer Extended Release Tablets
Therapy Bayer Caplets
Bufferin Caplets/Tablets
Vanquish Analgesic Caplets

*Common prescription products containing aspirin
or aspirin-like compounds*
Darvon Compund-65
Norgesic & Norgesic Forte Tablets
Disalcid Capsules/Tablets
Percodan/Oxycodone and Aspirin
Easprin Tablets
Robaxisal Tablets
Empirin with Codeine Tablets
Salflex Tablets
Fiorinal Capsules/Tablets
Talwin Compound Tablets
Lortab ASA Tablets
Trilisate Tablets/Liquid
Magsal Tablets
Mono-Gesic Tablets

Common nonprescription products containing ibuprofen
Advil Caplets/Tablets
Advil Cold/Sinus Caplets
Bayer Select Ibuprofen Pain Relief
Formula Caplets
Dristan Sinus Caplets
Sine-Aid IB
Haltran Tablets
Midol IB Tablets
Motrin IB Caplets/Tablets

*Common nonprescription products containing naproxen
sodium*
Aleve Caplets/Tablets

Prescription products containing naproxen/naproxen sodium
Naprosyn Suspension/Tablets
Anaprox/Anaprox DS Tablets

Prescription products containing ibuprofen
Motrin Tablets
Children's Advil Suspension
Children's Motrin Suspension

Vitamin supplements to avoid
Vitamin E
Alpha-omega vitamin supplements

a pharmacist when the ingredients of a drug are unknown. Before discontinuing any medication, the physician who prescribed the medication should be notified.

Wound healing

Glucocorticoids, antiplatelet agents, anticoagulants, and nicotine should also be discounted before surgery. Nicotine has been shown to be an important cause of flap necrosis [5]. Patients must discontinue use at least 1 week preoperatively and not restart until 2 to 4 days postoperatively. All patients should be encouraged to stop smoking regardless of impending surgery.

Drug interactions

Nurses should beware of the geriatric populations who use a wide variety of systemic medications, and should ensure that a careful screening of all medications is performed. This section discusses some of the more common medications and their systemic affects.

Diuretics

Altered electrolytes, in combination with epinephrine, may cause unwanted cardiac arrhythmias. Blood electrolytes (sodium, potassium) should be assessed preoperatively. Diuretics should be withheld on the preoperative morning because of potential volume and electrolyte imbalances.

Antidepressants

Phenothiazine and tricyclic medications may potentate cardiostimulatory effects of epinephrine. These agents should be discontinued 1 to 2 weeks before elective surgery when epinephrine is used. The patient's psychiatrist should always be consulted and the risk of withdrawal versus intraoperative risks should be weighed.

Propranolol

Propranolol can cause malignant hypertension and reflux bradycardia. The amount of epinephrine diluted in Xylocaine should be considered in patients taking beta-blockers.

Herbal medications

Patients often fail to disclose the herbal medications they are taking. Commonly used herbal medications, such as Echinacea, ephedra, garlic, gingko, ginseng, kava, St. John's wort, valerian, and vitamin E, may cause direct drug interactions, alteration of the action of drug, and alteration of the absorption, distribution, metabolism, and elimination of drugs. Gingko should be discontinued at least 7 days preoperatively because it may inhibit platelet-activating factor, causing an increased bleeding potential [5]. Vitamin E also may thin the blood, causing increased bleeding during surgical procedures.

Finally

Patients must be questioned about all medications they are taking, including prescriptions, inhalers, and herbal and nonprescription drugs. Patients are often not fully informed about which medications they are taking and why. They should be asked to provide a complete list of all medications. If an unfamiliar medication is encountered, a pharmacist or drug reference book should be consulted to identify product information. Many drugs are cross-referenced under brand and generic name listings that can confuse patients and staff.

Psychosocial data

Age, sex, marital status, occupation, and family and social support systems are important to review, because they provide insight into the patient's coping skills and the potential effect of surgery on the patient's lifestyle. Support systems, such as homecare and rehabilitation services, may need to be arranged before surgery. Family members may need to be available to accompany the patient home, depending on the extent of the surgery and type of anesthetic used (ie, general versus local).

Past medical history

All past medical conditions, treatment, and current health status must be reviewed.

Past family history

History of any blood relatives who had a problem with an anesthetic, malignant hypothermia, sickle cell, porphyria, or cholinesterase deficiency should be reviewed. All of these factors directly affect patients receiving general anesthesia.

Past surgical history

Past surgeries, reason for surgery, and any postsurgery complications must be reviewed. Patients should be questioned as to previous untoward experiences with local or general anesthetics.

Preoperative testing

Further evaluation or testing may be required, depending on the patient's underlying medical condition and the planned procedure. Tests may be recommended, such as hemoglobin levels if the patient has a history of anemia or is a women aged 45 or younger who is still menstruating; potassium levels if the patient is taking diuretics; chest radiograph if the patient has signs of unstable cardiopulmonary disease; or ECG if the patient has risk factors such as unstable coronary syndromes.

Physical examination

A physical examination may include height, weight, vital signs (eg, blood pressure, pulse, respiratory rate), cardiovascular assessment (eg, heart rate, rhythm, heart sounds), and pulmonary assessment (eg, breath sounds, cough, sputum, skin color) [21].

Preassessment screening: infectious diseases

To decrease the risk and spread of infectious diseases, some clinics may screen for methicillin-resistant staphylococcus aureus and vancomycin-resistant enterococci. All patient care activities should be performed consistent with the principles and practice of body substance precautions. Infection Prevention and Control Manuals should be located in each surgical suite. Screening for hepatitis A, B, or C and HIV is also at the discretion of the clinic. Universal precautions should be used in all surgical suites to decrease contact and spread of all diseases.

Initial preassessment summary

Nursing management in the initial assessment of the surgical patient identifies the patient's physical and psychological status. Patients should understand all risks and benefits and be fully informed as to anticipated surgical outcomes before undergoing surgery. Nurses should assess whether patients seem agitated or have unrealistic expectations about the surgical outcome. Any disabilities or physical limitations that may interfere with the intraoperative or postoperative phase of surgery should be documented. Allergies (including food, latex, and medications), current medications, blood pressure abnormalities, past or current major illnesses, past surgeries, seizures, use of tobacco, history of cardiac or respiratory disease, and a family or past history of anesthetics reactions should be noted in the patient's medical record. Referrals to specialists and presurgical tests should be completed and noted so that results will be available on the day of surgery.

Preassessment: day of surgery

At admission for surgery, a brief review and update of the patient's assessment data, including medications, physical status, and baseline blood pressure, respiration, and pulse, should be recorded in the patient's medical record. Allergies and the completed preoperative checklist should be included in the medical record. All past tests, including blood work, chest radiograph, and ECG, should be available. The patient's physical status must be stable before surgery. During the preassessment admission process, the nurse can review the proposed surgery with the patient. This final assessment is an opportune time to review postoperative expectations and provide the patient time to ask further questions [22].

Summary

With the increase in office-based surgery, the demand for experienced well-trained nurses will also increase. The practice of nursing in an office-based surgical suite requires specialized knowledge and clinical skills to offer continued well-informed care to patients. Standards and policies surrounding patient selection, personnel, preassessment protocols, preoperative testing, and maintenance of an accredited surgical suite should exist in all offices. A thorough evaluation of a patient's health status should be reviewed and documented before all surgical procedures. Nurses should never underestimate the importance and value of meeting the highest standards possible for patients, even when employed outside of the hospital setting.

The American Nurses Association Standards of Clinical Nursing Practice compel all nurses to acquire and maintain current knowledge and competency in nursing practice to ensure patients receive the best care offered while under their care [23]. All patients undergoing surgery (whether a punch biopsy, Mohs surgery, or more complex procedures such as liposuction) require a surgical preassessment of their health history to reduce risks. Patients must receive information about all possible complications and risks before surgery to make an informed consent. Nurses can make a positive difference in the surgical outcome of patients by being educated and informed about the steps required to ensure the safety and reduce the anxiety of office-based surgical patients. Patient safety is vital to ensure that the continued growth of office-based practices is preserved and, more importantly, that quality patient care is never compromised in the process.

Surgical preassessment benefits patients, physicians, and nurses through not only improving surgical outcomes and patient satisfaction but also ensuring patient safety.

References

[1] Dermatology Nurses Association (DNA). Annual membership statistics, 2006. Pitman (NJ): DNA.

[2] Anello S. Office-based surgery: advantages and disadvantages, and the nurse's role. Plast Surg Nurs 2002;22:107–11.
[3] Horton J, Reece E, Broughton G, et al. Patient safety in the office-based setting. Plast Reconstr Surg 2006;117(4):61e–80e.
[4] Byrd HS, Barton FE, Orentstein HH, et al. Safety and efficacy in an accredited outpatient plastic surgery facility: a review of 5316 consecutive cases. Plast Reconstr Surg 2003; 112(2):636–41.
[5] Rauscher G, Mancchshana B, Schwartz R. 2005. Preoperative evaluation and management. Available at: www.emedicine.com/derm/topic819.htm. Assessed August 16, 2006.
[6] Patton CM. Preoperative nursing assessment of the adult patient. Semin Perioper Nurs 1999; 8(1):42–7.
[7] Duffy SQ, Farley DE. Patterns of decline among inpatient procedures. Public Health Rep 1995;110(6):674–81.
[8] Leader S, Moon M. Medicare trends in ambulatory surgery. Health Aff 1989;8(1):158–70.
[9] Kozak LJ, Owings MF. Ambulatory and inpatient procedures in the United States, 1995. Vital Health Stat 13 1998;135:1–116.
[10] American Society for Aesthetic Plastic Surgery. Quick facts: highlights of the ASAP's 2005. Statistics on cosmetic surgery. Available at: www.surgery.org/press/statistics.php. Accessed August 15, 2006.
[11] Tuleya S. A status report: dermatological surgery. Skin Aging 2002;10(5):48–9.
[12] 2005 ASAPS News Release. Cosmetic plastic surgery statistics, Available at: www.cosmeticplasticsurgerystatistics.com/statistics.html. Assessed August 15, 2006.
[13] Aasi S. Complications in dermatologic surgery. Arch Dermatol 2003;139:213–4.
[14] Muliira J. The Nation wide nursing shortage in USA. Work force trends in public health. 2006. Available at: http://www.case.edu/med/epidbio/mphp439/Nursing_Shortage.htm. Accessed August 18, 2006.
[15] Bitar G, Mullis W, Jacobs W, et al. Safety and efficacy of office-based surgery with monitored anesthesia care/sedation in 4778 consecutive plastic surgery procedures. Plast Reconstr Surg 2003;111(1):150–6, B.
[16] University of Pennsylvania. 2002. Study of US nurses finds young leaving profession; nurse shortage may reach crisis sooner than thought. Available at: http://upenn.edu?reserachatpenn/article.php/435&soc. Accessed August 8, 2006.
[17] Bruce P. Off-site preadmission unit supports hospital ambulatory surgical unit. J Anesth Nurs 1993;8(4):262–9.
[18] Hammons T, Piland N, Small S, et al. Ambulatory patient safety. What we know and need to know. J Ambul Care Manage 2003;26(1):63–82. Available at: www.outpatientsurgery.net/2002/0503/f2,shtml. Accessed August 8, 2006.
[19] American Association of Nurse Anesthetists. Standards for office-based anesthesia practice. Available at: www.aana.com. Accessed August 23, 2006.
[20] Fuller J, Schaller-Ayers J. Health assessment: a nursing approach. In: Jarvic C, editor. Nursing assessment; physical assessment. 2nd edition. Philadelphia: J.B. Lippincott; 1994. p. 702.
[21] Rogers B. Perioperative nursing. In: Nettina SM, editor. Lippincott manual of nursing practice. 8th edition. Philadelphia: Lippincott-Raven Publishers; 2006. p. 104–13.
[22] Institute for Clinical Systems Improvement (ICSI). Preoperative evaluation. Bloomington (MN): institute for clinical systems improvement; 2003. p. 43. Available at: www.guideline.gov/summary/summary.aspx?doc-id. Accessed October 5, 2006.
[23] American Nurses Association (ANA). Standards of clinical nursing practice. 2nd edition. Washington (DC): ANA; 1998.

ELSEVIER
SAUNDERS

Nurs Clin N Am 42 (2007) 379–392

NURSING
CLINICS
OF NORTH AMERICA

The Role of Sentinel Node Biopsy in Patients with Cutaneous Melanoma

Lakshi M. Aldredge, RN, MSN, ANP

*Dermatology Service, Portland VA Medical Center, P.O. Box 1034,
Portland, OR 97207, USA*

The role of sentinel lymph node biopsy (SLNB) as a prognostic indicator in melanoma patients has been controversial in the fields of surgical oncology and dermatology for decades. This minimally invasive surgical technique was introduced in 1990 for diagnosing melanoma lymphatic metastases [1] and has been deemed the standard of surgical care of cutaneous malignant melanoma by the World Health Organization and the Sunbelt Melanoma Clinical Trial [2]. Its usefulness as a prognostic indicator of metastases led to expanded applications for breast, colon, gastric, esophageal, head and neck, thyroid, and lung cancers [1]. The National Comprehensive Cancer Network and the American Society of Clinical Oncology endorse sentinel node biopsy as the preferred staging procedure for breast cancer [3] where it has been widely used.

Preliminary findings from the first major prospective randomized trial on SLNB, the multicenter selective lymphadenectomy trial-1 (MSLT-1), were published this past fall and provide the best data supporting the use of this procedure in patients who have intermediate thickness melanoma [4]. This article first provides an overview of cutaneous melanoma and staging methods and treatment modalities. A brief study of the lymphatic system and the SLNB procedure are reviewed, followed by a discussion of its usefulness in patients who have melanoma, including risks and benefits. This article also discusses nursing considerations for patients undergoing the procedure, and patient education tips. Lastly, future indications for SLNB and new prognostic indicators for melanoma are discussed.

Melanoma

Melanoma is a malignant tumor arising within the melanocytes of the skin [5]. Therefore, they are typically black or brown, but occasionally

E-mail address: lakshi.aldredge@va.gov

0029-6465/07/$ - see front matter © 2007 Elsevier Inc. All rights reserved.
doi:10.1016/j.cnur.2007.06.001   *nursing.theclinics.com*

some will stop producing pigment and appear skin-colored, pink, or reddish purple [6]. The incidence of cutaneous melanoma has continued to markedly rise worldwide in the past decades. It is the sixth most common cancer in the United States, is the most common of all cancers in young women aged 25 to 29 years, and is second only to breast cancer in women aged 30 to 34 years [6]. It is among the most common types of cancer in young adults, and is therefore a very pressing and public concern. Up to one fifth of patients diagnosed with a cutaneous melanoma will develop metastatic disease, which usually results in death [5]. Early diagnosis and determining risk factors for metastases are therefore imperative to obtain the best outcomes for patients.

Melanoma has four subtypes that are based on their growth patterns: superficial spreading melanoma, nodular melanoma, lentigo maligna, and acral lentiginous melanoma [5]. Of these, nodular melanoma is the only invasive type and is the most aggressive [6]. However, identifying the subtype alone is not useful in determining prognosis but must be considered along with other staging methods.

Microstaging

When a patient is diagnosed with a cutaneous melanoma after a skin biopsy, the single most important predictive factor in staging is determining the thickness of the primary lesion, otherwise known as *Breslow depth* or *thickness* (Table 1) [5]. It is measured in millimeters from the top of the granular level of the epidermis to the deepest point of tumor penetration [5]. In addition to looking at the depth of penetration, the lesion is usually assessed for ulceration, meaning that the epidermis on top of the melanoma is not intact. Breslow thickness, along with the presence or absence of ulceration, is considered one of the most significant factors in predicting progression of melanoma [6].

Another factor used in microstaging a melanoma is the Clark's level of invasion, which measures the depth of melanoma penetration from the epidermis to subcutaneous fat, and ranges from level I (the epidermis) to level V (the subcutaneous fat) (Table 2) [6]. Other helpful clues to determining prognosis include identifying the presence of tumor-infiltrating lymphocytes, vascular invasion, and microscopic satellites [5]. Unfortunately, no

Table 1
Breslow thickness scale[a]

In situ	Melanoma is confined to the epidermis
<1 mm	Very thin tumors
1 mm–2 mm	Thin tumors
2 mm–4 mm	Intermediate thickness tumors
>4 mm	Thick melanomas

[a] Distance from uppermost epidermis to deepest point of melanoma tumor penetration.

Table 2
Clark's level of invasion[a]

Level I	Occupies only the epidermis
Level II	Penetrates to the layer just below the epidermis (papillary dermis)
Level III	Fills the papillary dermis and impinges on the next level (reticular dermis)
Level IV	Penetrates into the reticular or deep dermis
Level V	Invades the subcutaneous fat

[a] Number of layers of skin penetrated by the melanoma tumor from epidermis to fat.

reliable immunohistological markers or stains help differentiate benign melanocytic tumors from melanomas at the cellular level. Likewise, no blood tests are specific for detecting melanomas, and most imaging studies are only useful in detecting invasive or metastatic disease. Therefore, this discussion focuses on the most important staging factor, Breslow thickness.

Breslow thickness was initially noted in the following gradations: 1 mm or less (very thin tumors), 1 to 2 mm (thin tumors), 2 to 4 mm, and 4 mm or more [5]. However, the following limits have been found to be more useful: less than 1 mm (thin), 1 to 2 mm (intermediate), and 2 to 4 mm (thick). Melanomas that are in situ are confined to the epidermis and can be easily and completely removed with wide excision, and therefore are not lesions that are considered for SLNB. Because categorizing thickness after 4 mm has not been found to be useful, size larger than 4 mm has become the end point for thickness categorization.

Although thickness is essential in staging melanoma, the single most important prognostic indicator for patients who have melanoma is the involvement of regional lymph nodes [7].

Staging

The American Joint Committee on Cancer (AJCC) developed a classification system that is now the standard used for staging melanoma [5]. Determining the stage of melanoma is imperative to establishing if local, regional, or distant metastatic disease is present. These factors strongly correlate with prognosis and determine the appropriate path of treatment (Table 3).

The AJCC classification system considers the melanoma based on Breslow depth, regional lymph node involvement, and distant metastases [5]. Revisions in the staging system over the past decade now also consider the presence of microscopic ulceration, local recurrence, satellite disease and in-transit metastases, the number of positive lymph nodes, the presence of elevated serum lactate dehydrogenase, and the site of distant metastases [5]. The grouping for staging melanoma ranges from stage 0 (5-year survival, 95%) to stage IV (5-year survival, 7.5%–11%).

Although staging is the most important factor in determining prognosis, this discussion focuses on tumor thickness and the subsequent treatment pathways.

Table 3
Major factors in staging melanoma

Type of melanoma	Superficial spreading, nodular, lentigo maligna and acral lentiginous melanoma
Localized, regional, or distant disease	In situ, regional lymph node involvement, distant metastases
Thickness (Breslow depth): ≤1 mm, 1–2 mm, 2–4 mm, >4 mm	Measures the distance between the uppermost layer of epidermis to the deepest point of tumor penetration
Ulceration	Epidermis on top of melanoma is not intact
Clark's level of invasion: levels 1–5	Number of layers of skin penetrated by the tumor (epidermis to fat)
Regression	Presence of lymphocytes near tumor (may indicate that this was a larger tumor initially)

Prognosis

Patients who have local disease and no nodal or distant metastases and are noted to have thin melanomas (≤1 mm) have a very good prognosis (5-year survival, >90%) [8]. These patients are treated with wide local excision (WLE) of the primary tumor. In patients who have thicker primary melanomas (>1 mm), prognosis is less certain, especially when no evidence is seen of local or regional metastases [4]. These patients are typically managed with two approaches: (1) WLE of the primary melanoma with elective lymph node dissection (ELND) or (2) clinical observation after WLE of the primary site with complete lymph node dissection (CLND) after regional lymph node involvement becomes clinically detectable [4]. The removal of lymph nodes, either at WLE or after noting palpable nodes, is not without risk. This procedure can be painful and result in complications such as lymphedema, which is a difficult condition to manage.

In 1998, the World Health Organization performed a study comparing ELND against observation and CLND [4]. The study suggested a slight outcome benefit for ELND patients who had occult nodal melanoma over those who developed regional lymph node involvement during observation [4]. However, the ELND procedure (which removes all relevant regional nodes) is a radical treatment that overtreats 80% of patients who have no nodal involvement who may then develop significant complications postprocedure [4]. Alternatively, patients who underwent delayed lymph node dissection after observation who did not have nodal disease were spared the morbidity associated with CLND. However, those who developed occult nodal disease after observation and CLND developed larger tumors in individual nodes [4].

In 1990, Morton and colleagues developed a procedure for lymphatic mapping to identify the lymphatic pathway from the primary melanoma, target nodal basin and the initial draining lymph node, or *sentinel node* [8]. This procedure has rapidly become the preferred method of determining the histopathologic status of regional lymph nodes [8]. The actual sentinel lymph node (SLN) procedure is discussed in greater detail in a later section.

The lymphatic system

The lymphatic system is part of the body's immune system, helping to fight off infection and cancers. All tissues are surrounded by lymph fluid, which drains into lymphatic vessels and lymph nodes throughout the body [6]. Lymph nodes are found in clusters throughout the body and filter the lymph fluid and its contaminants, such as bacteria. When a lymph node is in the process of filtering contaminated lymph fluid, it must produce additional white cells to fight off infection. This swelling is usually palpated by the provider and is an early indication of illness. Not all swollen lymph nodes indicate severe illness but may represent a recent illness. Lymph nodes can return to normal size after days without any treatment. Persistently swollen lymph nodes, however, can indicate more serious illness and should be evaluated.

Lymph nodes in the neck drain the head, axillary nodes drain the arms, and leg lymphatic drainage is filtered through nodes in the groin. Many smaller nodes are located along the pathway, but these are the primary areas examined and palpated during physical examination. When a patient has a melanoma in the arm, for example, the primary lymphatic drainage system would be in the axillary region and this would be the focal area to assess for metastases.

Cutaneous melanomas are believed to metastasize through the lymphatic system by first traveling to the nearest lymph node (sentinel node), then through the regional nodes, and eventually through the distant lymphatic system [9]. Therefore, the first stop in the pathway of metastases is typically the sentinel node. However, distal metastases can occur without regional lymph node involvement.

Sentinel lymph node biopsy

Procedure

SLNB is a procedure in which a sample of tissue is removed from the first lymph node in the pathway from the primary tumor to the nodal basin. The procedure is performed after skin biopsy has determined the diagnosis of melanoma and the patient has undergone tumor staging. The procedure is performed in an outpatient setting, usually in an operative suite. The surgeon injects a blue marker dye or radioactive substance called a *tracer* near the site of the primary melanoma (Figs. 1 and 2). The radiation dose in the tracer is equal to that of a standard radiograph [10] and is safe. The radioactive tracer is visualized using radiographic imagery known as *lymphoscintigraphy* in which the surgeon is able to see where the tracer

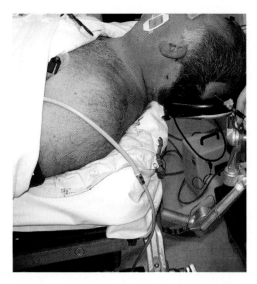

Fig. 1. Melanoma patient prepared for sentinel lymph node biopsy.

and dye have traveled through the lymphatic system to the nearest lymph node, thus identifying the sentinel node (Fig. 3). The surgeon may also use a handheld Geiger counter to determine the location of the sentinel node. This instrument emits an audible tone, revealing the exact location of the sentinel node [11] and any other nodes that may be positive. Once the sentinel node is identified, the surgeon makes a small incision over the lymph node area and removes the sentinel node. The presence of the blue

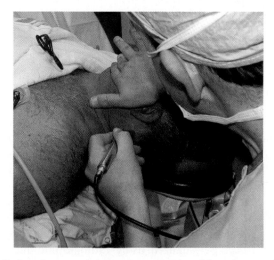

Fig. 2. Radioactive tracer is injected near the site of the primary melanoma.

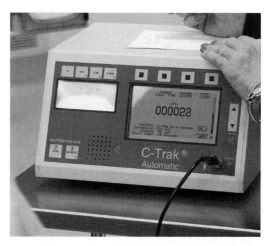

Fig. 3. Geiger counter used to detect radioactive tracer injected near primary melanoma site.

dye at the sentinel node site confirms the lymphatic flow to the sentinel node. Most surgeons will remove all nodes that contain blue dye and any nodes that contain at least 10% of the radioactivity of the "hottest" node.

After the sentinel node is removed, the surgeon closes the incisions with a few sutures. The sentinel node is then sent for histopathologic testing to determine if the melanoma has spread to the lymph nodes. A dressing is applied at the biopsy site and the patient returns in 1 to 2 weeks for suture removal.

If the SLN is found to be positive for tumor cells, other nodes in the basin are probably affected and usually removed using CLND [4]. If the sentinel node is negative, other nodes in the basin will probably not be positive and usually no further surgical intervention is warranted [4].

Effectiveness

SLNB has been shown to be an effective and efficient method of identifying and removing the sentinel node. A report published by Landi and Landi [2] showed that lymphoscintigraphy and interoperative mapping using blue dye and radiographic tracer was successful almost 100% in identifying sentinel nodes. The ability to correctly identify tumor cells in the sentinel node has also been successful. Balch and Cascinelli [3] reported that in a trial conducted by Morton and colleagues, the rate of false-negative results on biopsy was only 3.4%. The complications from the SLNB procedure were believed to be minor and occurred in approximately 10% of patients [1].

Although it is safe and effective, SLNB is a difficult procedure to master despite its widespread use. Morton and colleagues worked hard to perfect the procedure in patients who had melanoma. Their initial reports identified the SLN in only 81% of patients [1]. During the next 58 cases, their success rate increased from 96% to 100% [1], showing that surgeon experience is directly related to the successful identification of the SLN [1].

Risks

SLNB has proven to be a cost-effective method to accurately determine regional lymph node metastases in patients who have melanoma. Although it is a simple outpatient procedure, it is not without risk. Adverse effects include:

- Excessive bleeding at the site of lymph node biopsy
- Pain or numbness at the site of lymph node biopsy
- Infection
- Edema at the site of removal, which can occur immediately after the procedure or even months or years later (lymphedema)
- Nerve damage at the site of biopsy
- Anaphylaxis in 1% of patients from the blue dye used during the procedure [1]

In addition, in rare cases an SLNB may not provide a definite diagnosis and a more complicated surgical procedure known as an *open lymph node biopsy* may be necessary.

SLNB should not be undertaken if the prognostic information will not change the course of clinical management, such as in extremely elderly patients or those who have more significant comorbid conditions [1]. SLNB is not indicated in patients who have previous histologically confirmed lymph node involvement or underwent previous extensive surgery at the primary melanoma site [1].

Although some experts have questioned whether removing a positive SLN can be deleterious to the immune system, no published data have supported this [4]. In addition, some experts have speculated that SLNB can contribute to in-transit metastasis, but studies have refuted this claim also [4].

Benefits

Since 1990, the use of SLNB greatly increased and many patients have been spared the risks of CLND. Repeated studies have shown that if the SLN is tumor-free, melanoma is probably not present in the other lymph nodes in the regional basin [4]. Therefore, the need for ELND or CLND may be deferred in lieu of further observation, sparing patients the risks of these procedures, which can result in pain, lymphedema, or nerve damage. The ability of SLNB to identify early disease and its cost-effectiveness also make it an appealing alternative to CLND. Patients can also appreciate the simplicity of the outpatient procedure, low complication rate, and speed of recovery.

In summary, the primary reasons for advocating SLNB are (1) to minimize the morbidity associated with other lymph node assessment methods

(CLND), (2) to identify the most appropriate therapeutic surgical procedure or treatment pathway based on sentinel node status, and (3) to improve the accuracy of SLN assessment [1].

Nursing considerations for patients undergoing sentinel lymph node biopsy for melanoma

The diagnosis of melanoma is devastating to most patients. They usually associate this term with metastatic disease and death. Although the physician or practitioner is responsible for notifying the patient of the diagnosis, often the nurse must provide further clarification of what this diagnosis means for the patient. The nurse must understand the types of melanoma and staging levels of melanoma, and should reassure the patient and explain that further testing will help determine the treatment plan. Box 1 lists areas in which nurses should have knowledge when dealing with patients undergoing SLNB.

Patient teaching

Patients should be counseled thoroughly about the risks and benefits of the procedure and all pre- and postoperative teaching. It is important to educate patients about excessive bleeding at the site; pain or numbness at the site; infection; edema at the site of removal, which can occur immediately after the procedure or even months or years later (lymphedema); and nerve damage at the site of biopsy [12]. Rarely, an SLNB may not provide a definite diagnosis and an open lymph node biopsy may be necessary. Patients should also be told that they may notice a bluish discoloration around the cancer site from the injected dye, which will also cause their urine to turn green for about 24 hours.

Providing verbal and written instructions gives patients the opportunity to ask questions and a tangible resource to share with family members and friends.

Clinical studies and controversy regarding sentinel lymph node biopsy in melanoma

After the initial introductory reports from Morton and colleagues, SLNB became widely used, with subsequent reports showing its value in predicting relapse-free survival in patients who have melanoma [4].

The Stanford Study

The Stanford Study evaluated the investigators' experience with SLNB over a 7-month period and confirmed previous findings that SLN status

---

Box 1. Considerations for nurses when dealing with patients undergoing sentinel lymph node biopsy

- SLNB is usually performed as an outpatient procedure and takes approximately 60 to 90 minutes
- Medical history should include information about allergies to medications and whether patients are taking any blood-thinning agents that can cause excessive bleeding during or after the procedure
- Patients who are anxious may require a sedative before the procedure
- Nurses should follow pre-, intra-, and postoperative procedures for monitoring patients when general anesthesia is used
- Patients may need to remove a portion or all of their clothing and be positioned accordingly
- After the procedure, patients will have a pressure dressing and may experience minimal pain and a small amount of drainage from the biopsy site
- Nurses should provide patient education that includes biopsy site dressing information, signs and symptoms of infection, and pain management education (although pain is usually minimal)
- Nurses should ensure that the patient has a ride home, because they may still feel the effects of procedure sedation
- Nurses should follow-up with a phone call to ensure that patients are not experiencing any side effects from the procedure

---

correlates with relapse-free survival rates [4]. Of 260 cases, 39 of AJCC stage I and II melanoma showed sentinel node positivity (15%) [4]. In patients who had negative SLNs, the recurrence rate (ie, false-negative rate) was 4.5% [4], which was less than that found by Morton and colleagues in earlier studies. In the Stanford Study, 31 of the 39 patients who had positive SLNs underwent SLNB; 7 of these were found to have nonnodal metastases [4]. The study also showed that 46% of patients who had positive SLNs experienced recurrence versus 14% of patients who had negative SLNs [4]. In addition, the patients who had negative SLNs had a 17-month median relapse-free survival compared with 8 months in those who had positive SLNs [4].

Although the Stanford Study showed the usefulness of SLNB in predicting relapse-free survival, it also noted that recurrence rates were different for patients who had thicker tumors (Breslow thickness >2 mm) [4]. In these patients, 53% of patients who had positive SLNs experienced recurrence compared with 24% of those who had negative SLNs [4]. In further analysis, other clinical and pathologic features were correlated with SLN positivity, including Breslow thickness, ulceration, gender, age, and site [4]. Truncal location, Breslow thickness, male gender, and histologic ulceration were strongly associated with SLN positivity, with ulceration noted to be the most predictive of these factors [4].

The Multicenter Selective Lymphadenectomy Trial-1 clinical trial

In 1994, Morton and colleagues at the John Wayne Cancer Institute began a study to determine the therapeutic benefit of SLNB and the accuracy of the technique on a worldwide basis, known as the Multicenter Selective Lymphadenectomy Trial-1 (MSLT-1) [13]. This study randomized 2001 patients who had Breslow thickness less than 1.2 mm, 1.2 to 3.5 mm, and more than 3.5 mm into two arms: wide local excision (WLE) and observation, or WLE and SLNB, followed by immediate CLND if the sentinel node was positive [4]. The group planned to have five outcome analyses, and in late 2004, the third interim analysis reported interesting data that affected patients who had melanoma of Breslow thickness between 1.2 and 3.5 mm [4]. The report noted that the absence or presence of tumor in the SLN was the most predictive survival factor for patients undergoing SLNB, with a reported 88% 5-year survival for 944 patients who had negative nodes and 71% for 215 who had positive nodes [4]. In addition, the patients who had positive SLNs had a 27.2% melanoma-specific mortality rate compared with 9.8% for those who had negative SLNs [4].

Metastatic disease was identified in 215 patients who underwent SLNB (18%), and 18% of those undergoing observation after WLE experienced nodal recurrence [4]. Therefore, 82% of patients had a tumor-free SLN and 82% observed after WLE have not developed regional metastases [4]. The 5-year disease-free survival rate was 78% for patients who underwent SLNB versus 73% for those treated with WLE plus observation [4]. Patients who had CLND after a positive SLNB showed a statistically significant higher 5-year survival rate (71%) compared with those who were deferred until they had clinically detectable nodes (55%) [4]. Disease-free survival was also higher in the positive SLNB plus CLND group [4].

These interim results from the MSLT-1 study provide the first evidence of survival benefits associated with SLNB versus WLE and observation in the management of intermediate-thickness melanoma [4].

Future indications for sentinel lymph node biopsy in patients who have melanoma

The recent interim results from the MSLT-1 study, which show survival benefit associated with SLNB for intermediate-thickness melanoma, have led experts to question the use of SLNB for thick and thin melanomas. An excellent summary by Cochran and Swetter [4] in *The Melanoma Letter* presents these questions as areas for further study.

With melanomas of more than 4 mm thickness, despite the risk for hematogenous spread, SLNB may be recommended to help with local and regional control of disease (bulky nodal disease is associated with higher morbidity and poorer quality of life) [4]. In addition, determining nodal involvement in thick melanomas may upstage patients to stage III, permitting acceptance into clinical trials or consideration of adjuvant therapy [4].

Patients who have thinner melanomas may wish to undergo SLNB for reassurance. The interim results of the MSLT-1 did not show that SLNB offered a survival advantage for patients who had melanomas less than 1.2 mm [4]. However, in a recent retrospective study of 148 patients who underwent SLNB for clinically localized melanoma less than 1 mm, Ranieri and colleagues [14] concluded that SLNB is a significant predicator of outcome. In this study, 6.5% of patients had positive SLNBs [14]. Disease-free survival and overall survival were significantly associated with SLNB status in these patients [14].

Although another study by Stizenberg and colleagues [8] noted that the incidence of positive SLNBs in thin melanomas (< 1.0 mm) was "considerable," the investigators were unable to identify predictors of SLNB positivity in these patients.

Future prognostic indicators for cutaneous melanoma

The SLNB status has become a highly valued prognostic indicator in patients who have melanoma. Although much work has been done with SLNB in melanoma, other studies are attempting to determine different methodologies that will determine SLN involvement in these patients.

In a 2005 study, 304 patients who had cutaneous melanoma who underwent SLNBs were also examined in situ by the same physician using high-resolution ultrasound [15]. Thirty-one patients had positive nodes, and ultrasound results in seven suggested metastatic disease [15]. The investigators determined that ultrasound was not a cost-effective methodology, because although it can detect metastatic disease deposits down to approximately 4.5 mm, most melanocytic deposits are smaller than that at initial staging [15].

Kell and colleagues [16] used a similar approach and assessed the value of positron emission tomography (PET)/CT in patients who had primary melanoma. Although this study did not support the use of PET/CT as a staging modality for detecting lymphatic metastases, it identified second occult malignancies in four (10.8%) patients undergoing therapy for melanoma.

Many studies are being conducted to determine future prognostic indicators for patients who have melanoma. Although SLNB is still an exceptional method for determining local/regional involvement, other more accurate, cost-effective, and efficient methods of determining prognosis for patients who have melanoma may exist.

Melanoma prevention

The most important way to prevent melanoma is to educate patients and the public about risk factors. Although genetics or a family history of melanoma is a key risk factor for determining whether an individual will develop melanoma, many other factors can increase the risk for developing melanoma. Exposure to natural sunlight or spending prolonged periods in the sun without protection can greatly increase chances of developing melanoma and other skin cancers. Tanning booths can definitely increase exposure to harmful ultraviolet A and B light. Peer pressure to look tan, especially for younger women, makes individuals more vulnerable to developing skin cancers, including melanoma. In fact, melanoma is the most common cancer found in women aged 25 to 29 years [6]. Previous history of blistering sunburns can also be a risk factor for the development of melanomas. Individuals who have a large number of moles and those who have a history of any type of skin cancer can be at increased risk for melanoma.

Nurses plays a key role in educating patients, their families, and the public about the risk factors for skin cancer. Avoiding prolonged sun exposure and tanning booths and wearing sun protection are excellent ways to protect oneself from developing melanomas.

Summary

The primary reasons for performing an SLNB are to (1) minimize the morbidity associated with lymph node assessment, (2) determine the most appropriate surgical procedure to be performed, and (3) improve the accuracy of nodal assessment and determine the level of nodal involvement [1]. Numerous past studies have confirmed the value of SLNB as a highly significant predictor of prognosis in melanomas of more than 1 mm thickness. Recent studies, however, have shown that SLNB is a significant predictor of outcome in intermediate and even thin melanomas, and should be considered a prognostic indicator for patients who have these lesions [14]. In addition, SLNB is a low-risk procedure that can identify patients who may not need to incur the cost or risks associated with ELND or CLND.

Acknowledgments

I would like to thank Heather Jones, RN, and Andrew Blauvelt, MD for their assistance in reviewing this article.

References

[1] Chen SL, Douglas MI, Randall PS, et al. Lymphatic mapping and sentinel node analysis: current concepts and applications. CA Cancer J Clin 2006;56:292–309.

[2] Landi G, Landi C. The sentinel node biopsy in melanoma patients. Dermatol Nurs 2001;13: 429–41.

[3] Balch CM, Cascinelli N. Sentinel-node biopsy in melanoma. N Engl J Med 2006;355:1370–1.

[4] Cochran AJ, Swetter SA. Sentinel lymph node biopsy 2006: the picture is becoming clearer. The Melanoma Letter 2006;24:1–4.

[5] Nestle FO, Kerl H, et al. Neoplasms of the skin: melanoma. In: Bolognia JL, Jorizzo JL, Rapini RP, editors. Dermatology. London: Mosby; 2003. p. 1789–811.

[6] Robins P, Perez M. Understanding melanoma: what you need to know. 2nd edition. New York: The Skin Cancer Foundation; 2005.

[7] Kuwarjerwala NK, Dwivedi A, Abbarah T, et al. Sentinel lymph node biopsy in patients with melanoma. Available at: www.emedicine.com.

[8] Stizenberg KAB, Groben PA, Stern SL, et al. Indications for lymphatic mapping and sentinel lymphadenectomy in patients with thin melanoma (Breslow thickness ≤1 mm). Ann Surg Oncol 2004;11:900–6.

[9] Perrot RE, Glass LF, Reintgen DS, et al. Reassessing the role of lymphatic mapping and sentinel lymphadenectomy in the management of cutaneous malignant melanoma. J Am Acad Dermatol 2003;49:567–88; quiz 589–92. Available at: www.home.mdconsult.com. Accessed January 2, 2007.

[10] What is lymphoscintigraphy? Available at: www.radiologyinfo.org. Accessed January 27, 2007.

[11] Sentinel lymph node biopsy. Available at: www.imaginis.com. Accessed January 4, 2007.

[12] Youngerman-Cole S. Sentinel lymph node biopsy. Available at: www.webmd.com. Accessed January 4, 2007.

[13] Morton DL, Thompson JF, Cochran AJ, et al. Sentinel-node biopsy or nodal observation in melanoma. N Engl J Med 2006;355:1307–17.

[14] Ranieri JM, Wagner JD, Wenck S, et al. The prognostic importance of sentinel lymph node biopsy in thin melanoma. Ann Surg Oncol 2006;13:927–32.

[15] Starritt EC, Uren RF, Scolyer RA, et al. Ultrasound examination of sentinel nodes in the initial assessment of patients with primary cutaneous melanoma. Ann Surg Oncol 2005; 12:18–23.

[16] Kell MR, Ridge JA, Joseph N, et al. PET CT imaging in patients undergoing sentinel node biopsy. Eur J Surg Oncol 2007 [Epub ahead of print].

NURSING CLINICS OF NORTH AMERICA

Nurs Clin N Am 42 (2007) 393–406

Nurse-Administered Laser in Dermatology

Heather Jones, RN, BSN

Dermatologic and Cutaneous Laser Surgery, Department of Dermatology, Oregon Health & Science University, 3303 SW Bond Avenue, Portland, OR 97229, USA

Laser technology in the dermatology setting is ever changing. With continuous advances come new considerations in nursing roles. Dermatology nurses must expand their knowledge and skills to ensure they keep in step with this rapidly changing technology. Laser is at the forefront of nursing roles and education in the dermatologic surgery setting, providing an opportunity for the nurse to have a new, exciting, and valuable role in patient care. Laser therapies that are available to patients have the potential to treat conditions ranging from cosmetic hair removal to bleeding vascular anomalies. Each year, increasing numbers of nurses are becoming competent in providing expert laser care to treat a variety of conditions in their patients. With appropriate training and experience, the nurse can play an essential role in administering much-needed quality care to patients in the dermatology setting, using the latest laser technology.

Laser technology and principles

For a nurse to provide the highest level of laser care for a patient, he or she first must understand the concepts associated with lasers and laser therapy. In 1917, Albert Einstein introduced the concept of the laser to the field of physics [1]. "Laser" is an acronym that stands for "light amplification by the stimulated emissions of radiation." All lasers operate on the same general principle: light amplification (generating more light) by the stimulated emission of radiation (by stimulating atoms with radiation, that is, light) [1].

Electron atoms normally are in a resting state. When an electron absorbs energy, it is raised to an excited state. This state is unstable, so the electron

E-mail address: joneshea@ohsu.edu

0029-6465/07/$ - see front matter © 2007 Elsevier Inc. All rights reserved. doi:10.1016/j.cnur.2007.07.001 *nursing.theclinics.com*

releases the absorbed energy to return to its normal, resting state. The released energy may be in the form of light. If an excited electron absorbs a pocket of energy, such as that in a photon (unit of light), two photons of light energy are released. The two photons of energy released have equal energy levels and move together in phase, producing light of the same frequency and wavelength. This process, called "stimulated emission of radiation," is repeated innumerable times, creating the high energy of a laser beam [1].

Laser light is monochromatic, highly coherent, and highly directional. Light from the sun or a light bulb is generally seen as white but contains many wavelengths of light that can be seen as different colors when white light is put through a prism. Laser light is different. It is generally monochromatic ("mono-," meaning "one"): it contains one specific wavelength of light. This wavelength of light can be seen as a single, intense color (red, blue, green, or yellow, depending on the laser) or can be invisible (ultraviolet or infrared). Lasers can and do produce more than one color. These colors, however, are discrete individual wavelengths of light, not the broad spectrum of sunlight or fluorescent light. The wavelengths in laser light can be thought of as organized. The photons of laser light all move in step with one another. Light from a light bulb, on the other hand, has wavelengths that are not nearly as organized, with most photons' waves traveling disorganized in several directions and running into one another. The coherent, organized property of laser light enables it to deliver a high amount of energy in a small beam. In the case of visible lasers, this high energy makes the laser beam very bright and intense because the photons in a laser beam travel parallel to each other instead of being scattered. For example, if a flashlight and a laser were directed simultaneously at a surface from the same distance, the flashlight would produce a wide, shining light, and the laser beam would produce a small, focused light [1].

All lasers consist of three basic elements: an optical or laser cavity, a lasting medium, and a power source. The optical cavity surrounds the lasting medium and consists of a reflective cavity with mirrors (one partially reflective) at each end facing each other. Light bounces back and forth between the mirrors, colliding into more and more atoms of the medium, creating high levels of energy. If one of the mirrors is made to be only partially transmitting (often as little as 1%), part of the light will escape out that end of the cavity. The escaped light forms the laser beam (Fig. 1) [2].

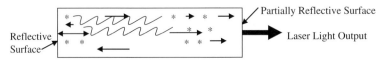

Chain reaction of electrons, creating laser light

Fig. 1. Chain reaction of electrons, creating laser light

The lasting medium within the laser often gives the laser its name and also supplies the electrons needed for the stimulated emission of radiation. The medium can be in the form of a gas (argon, copper vapor, krypton), a liquid (dye), a solid (ruby, erbium: yttrium-aluminum-garnet [YAG]), or a semiconductor (diode). The medium determines the wavelength of light that is emitted.

The power source that excites the electrons may come from a direct electric current, from a flash lamp, from radiofrequency waves, or from other laser energy [3].

When directed toward the skin, this light energy is absorbed by a specific chromophore. Chromophores are substances that absorb certain wavelengths of light. There are three identified chromophores: melanin, oxyhemoglobin, and water. Thermal (heat) damage to these chromophores removes the target entity (eg, a pigmented lesion such as a lentigo, which contains melanin, a vascular entity, such as a telangiectasia, which contains oxyhemoglobin, or skin that is to be resurfaced, which contains water). Specific wavelengths target these specific chromophores. The wavelength 595 nm, for example, targets the oxyhemoglobin within a blood vessel. Energy is taken up by the oxyhemoglobin, heating it to destroy the telangiectasia. In turn, the surrounding skin also could become heated. To reduce uptake of heat in the tissues around the vessel, and to prevent damage to the skin, the duration of the pulsed energy must be concise. This concept is called "selective photothermolysis." Selective photothermolysis refers to the technology where by laser light of sufficiently brief pulses causes selective thermal damage of microscopic chromophores, sparing the structures around them. The pulse duration of the laser must be shorter than the thermal relaxation time of the target chromophore. Thermal relaxation time is the time needed for half of the laser-induced heat to diffuse out of an absorbing chromophore [3]. To administer a safe and efficacious treatment, the nurse must ensure that the appropriate wavelength and pulse duration are used.

Types of lasers

Today nurses use several types of laser. As discussed previously, lasers have three main chromophores, melanin, oxyhemoglobin, and water. Although lasers may target more than one chromophore, lasers can be generally categorized based on their targets.

Lasers whose targets include oxyhemoglobin often are called "vascular lasers." Examples include argon, pulsed dye lasers (PDL), and neodymium: YAG lasers.

The argon laser, which uses argon gas for its medium, was the first laser used to treat port-wine stains (PWS) effectively. Unfortunately the laser produced nonselective damage, resulting in an increased risk for epidermal damage and hypertrophic scarring [3].

Other, more selective lasers, such as the PDL, have replaced the argon laser for many vascular lesions. In PDLs the light energy passes through a dye medium (liquid). PDLs were the first lasers developed based on the concept of photothermolysis. The 585- to 595-nm PDL with a 450-second pulse duration is used commonly for many vascular lesions today (Fig. 2). The laser effectively treats vascular conditions such as telangiectasia, PWS, poikiloderma of Civatte, and cherry angiomas [3]. PDL laser therapy leaves significant purpura of the skin (purple bruising at treatment site) that occurs as a result of the extravasations of the red blood cells from rupture of the vessels (Fig. 3). The purpura and accompanied swelling may last up to a week.

Short-pulsed (millisecond-pulsed green) neodymium:YAG lasers have a 532-nm wavelength that is well absorbed by hemoglobin. Pulse duration may range from 1 to 50 milliseconds. A longer pulse duration allows greater and more uniform heating of larger vessels. The lasers in this category include a diode-pumped Q-switched neodymium:YAG laser (CBDiode, Continuum Biomedical, Santa Clara, CA), a Q-switched potassium titanyl phosphate (KTP) laser (Aura KTP, Laserscope, San Jose, CA), a pulsed KTP laser (Versapulse, Lumenis, Santa Clara, CA), and a diode-pumped frequency doubled solid state laser (Diolite, IRIDEX Corporation, Mountain View, CA).

These lasers have been used successfully to treat adult hemangiomas, PWS, telangiectasia, and other vascular lesions. Leg veins can be treated effectively with lasers, but the optimal pulse duration for small leg veins has not been established in human studies with a neodymium:YAG laser [4]. The interlesional treatment of pediatric hemangiomas also has improved recently with the use of KTP or neodymium:YAG lasers [5,6].

With this group of vascular lasers, there is less chance of purpura, because these lasers allow slower heating of the vessels with less chance of vessel wall rupture. Overall improvement may take longer, or the patient

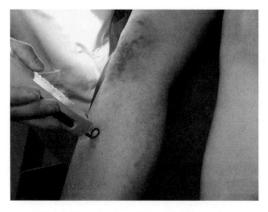

Fig. 2. Vascular laser to a port wine stain.

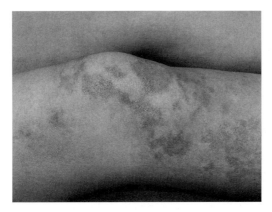

Fig. 3. Purpura immediately post vascular laser.

may require additional treatments to achieve clearing of vascular lesion. After treatment most patients develop mild redness and swelling that may last up to 24 hours.

Lasers that target melanin are used to treat conditions such as unwanted hair, tattoos, and pigmented lesions such as café au lait spots and lentigines.

An example of such a laser is the diode laser (semiconductor medium). Energy is emitted in the 800-nm wavelength. This laser has the ability to deliver energy deeply, targeting melanin and hemoglobin. This characteristic is preferential for hair removal and some small vessels. For hair removal, heat energy is transferred from the follicular matrix to the surrounding nonpigmented follicular epithelium and perifollicular dermis. The clinician seeks to induce perifolliculitis to achieve hair removal. Sufficient thermal injury to the follicle and its surrounding tissue results in miniaturization of follicles so that they become clinically unapparent for a variable duration of time. Differences in the content of melanin associated with differing stages in the hair cycle account for some follicles being more susceptible to photothermal injury than others [7]. Inflammation around the hair follicle may last 24 to 48 hours. The author's experience with hair removal indicates that optimal treatment regimens involve five or six treatments, with the patient being seen at 5- to 6-week intervals. The patient usually requires a touch-up treatment every 4 to 6 months to maintain the hair removal. Skin with the least amount of melanin in the skin and greatest amount in the follicle responds most quickly and achieves more lasting results. The 755-nm alexandrite laser (a solid-state laser using an alexandrite gem) also has shown results for hair removal but was the most painful in a study of lasers for hair removal [8]. The alexandrite laser, as well as the Q-switched ruby laser (which uses a ruby gem as a solid medium) can be used effectively for the treatment of pigmented lesions, tattoos, and hair. It is especially effective the removal of tattoos made with blue or black ink [9].

Intense pulsed light (IPL) is recent technology that uses a light source and, in fact, is not a laser at all. The IPL is an intense pulsed light that delivers light from 515 nm to 1200 nm at pulse durations ranging from 2 to 25 milliseconds in single, double, or triple pulses [3]. A coupling gel is applied to the skin before treatment to minimize epidermal damage and to increase the efficiency of light delivery to deeper structures. With the placement of cut-off filters that block the transmission of selected shorter wavelengths, specific wavebands can be generated from 515, 550, 570, and 590 to 1200 nm, making IPL useful for various types of vascular and pigmented conditions, including lentigines, telangiectasia, and unwanted hair [3] The IPL rarely leaves purpura or any evidence of treatment other than mild redness or swelling that resolves within several hours [3].

Dermatologic conditions and lasers

Port-Wine Stains and Hemangiomas

The PDL remains the treatment of choice for most PWS and hemangiomas within the author's clinic and within most literature. Flat and mildly hypertrophic PWS are best treated with the 585-nm PDL (450-second pulse) [3]. For significant improvement, multiple treatments often are needed, in some cases up to 15 to 20. Earlier studies showed that approximately 36% to 44% of the adult patients who have PWS experience 75% or more lightening, and 75% of patients experience at least 50% lightening of lesions after four treatments [3]. Clearing can depend on many factors, including the site, level of vasculature, and the patient's skin type. Facial PWS respond more quickly, followed by neck lesion and trunk and extremity lesions. Hemangiomas have been shown to involute spontaneously, so sometimes laser therapy can be controversial. Although superficial hemangiomas in the involution phase resolve spontaneously, early treatment seems to minimize enlargement of the tumor and can prevent complications such as bleeding and ulceration. Administering laser therapy also may hasten cosmetic improvement. Hemangiomas that are actively involuting generally respond quickly to the PDL, sometimes resolving in two to four treatments without anesthesia [3]. Patients are seen generally every 4 to 6 weeks for treatment of these vascular lesions.

Deep hemangiomas are more difficult to treat, and treatment must be titrated to the growth or stagnation of the lesion. When lesions are proliferating, some providers treat them more aggressively and at closer intervals, perhaps every 2 to 3 weeks. In some cases, the PDL may not absorb deeply enough to improve the deep component of the lesion. Lasers with longer wavelengths and pulse widths may be needed. Additionally, although the lesion may respond well, cavernous types of lesion may need debulking with surgery once the vascular component has been addressed.

Telangiectasia of the Face and Leg

Facial telangiectasia and spider angiomas on the body respond favorable to the PDL, IPL, and the neodymium:YAG laser, often with two or three treatments. The PDL will most certainly leave purpura, but it often requires fewer treatments.

Leg telangiectasia have shown to respond poorly to laser energy, and sclerotherapy continues to provide better results overall for patients. When leg vessels do respond, they tend to be more superficial and fine. A combination of laser and sclerotherapy often is recommended to achieve optimal results. Most promising results have been seen with the long-pulse (1.5-millisecond) 595-nm PDL, the 532-nm millisecond green-pulsed laser with a pulse width reaching 50 milliseconds, and the 800-nm diode laser [3]. When treating leg vessels, cooling is essential to help prevent burns. Hyperpigmentation is common for these superficial vessels and generally resolves in 4 to 6 weeks.

Scars

Scars always have been difficult to treat and remain so even with the best laser technology available. The patient should understand that improvement in the bulk and redness in the scar is all that can be anticipated. Results require multiple treatments and often adjuvant injection of steroid such as triamcinolone. Time will improve most scars, so the patient generally should be encouraged to be patient and wait the course of healing. When treatment is indicated, the 532-nm YAG laser or the 595-nm PDL commonly is used to soften the scar and reduce redness.

Hair

Hair removal has come a long way during the last decade, and hair now can be removed from patients of almost all skin types. Several types of laser have been used for hair removal. The alexandrite laser widely used for hair removal has been recognized as efficacious and generally safe. Blistering, crusting, and pigmentary alteration may occur in darker skin types even when cooling devices are used [8]. In a study performed by Lanigan [8] at the Birmingham Skin Center in 2003, the highest incidence of side effects was seen in patients who had darker skin treated with the long-pulsed ruby laser. With all hair-removal lasers, some of the laser light is absorbed by melanin in the skin as well as in the follicle, this absorption will be more significant in darker skin types and in suntanned skin. Thermal changes that occur can result in complications, including blistering, hypopigmentation, hyperpigmentation, and scar. Hyperpigmentation usually is reversible and results from the stimulation of melanin production from epidermal melanocytes similar to a UV-induced suntan. Hypopigmentation may be permanent and results from thermally induced destruction of melanocytes [8]. The diode laser can be used on dark-pigmented skin with positive outcomes.

Complications such as hypopigmentation or hyperpigmentation generally are transient, as seen in a study by Greppi [10]. Studies have used only small numbers of patients, so conscientious and slowly titrated treatments are judicious. With the new technology of the IPL, most skin types can now be treated with even less risk. Hyperpigmentation and hypopigmentation are very common risks associated with darker skin types. The authors have treated Fitzpatrick skin types IV and V successfully with the IPL, using the Lux Rs handpiece (Palomar Medical Technologies, Inc., Burlington, MA) with 100-millisecond pulse durations and prolonged cooling. Six to 10 treatments have been needed to achieve complete clearing, and some transient hypopigmentation has occurred.

Laser safety

With changes in laser technology come the dangers associated with laser light and laser energy. Because of the high degree of beam collimation, a laser serves as an almost ideal point source of intense light. A laser beam can produce retinal intensities greater than those from conventional light sources and even larger than those produced from directly viewing the sun. Permanent blindness can result [11,12]. Ocular damage is the most serious injury related to laser use and accounts for 73% of recorded laser incidents [3]. Laser light is extremely intense, and the eye may be exposed either directly in the laser beam's path or indirectly by a beam reflected by surfaces within the room. For lasers in the visible and near-infrared range, retinal damage is the main hazard; infrared lasers, which are well absorbed by water, may damage the cornea [3]. To avoid ocular damage, anyone working with a laser or present in a room where a laser is being operated should wear appropriate eye protection. Eyewear should be labeled clearly with the optical density and wavelength. If laser treatment is to be performed anywhere within the orbit of the eye, metal shields (contact lens) should be inserted over the patient's cornea. It is important to ensure that the appropriate size shield is selected for the patient. Goggles also should be placed outside the door at all times to ensure that anyone who may enter the room has access to protective eye wear. Additionally, appropriate signage should be placed outside the door, listing the wavelength of the specific laser and any other considerations. Within the author's clinical setting, lighted signs are connected to the power outlet of the laser. The laser cannot be powered without the "laser in use" sign being illuminated. This precaution helps improve the safety of the clinic by ensuring that persons outside the room know that a laser is being used appropriate precautions before entering. To prevent inadvertent firing of the laser, the system should be put in standby mode or turned off when not in use. Exposure to the solvents and organic dyes in dye laser systems is a potentially hazard, so the telephone numbers for chemical response teams should be posted. Fire is a risk with lasers, so an extinguisher should be kept immediately available.

Care must be taken to prevent inadvertent irradiation of adjacent skin, clothing, or personal effects. The surrounding field must be kept clear of flammable items, such as dry gauze, and of brightly reflective surfaces, such as surgical instruments. If surgical instruments are to be used, they should be ebonized so they are diffusely reflecting.

Staff should review laser competencies annually to demonstrate knowledge of all lasers within the practice. The nurse's specific roles in laser operation should be outlined clearly, including basic functions of on and off procedures, as well as direct patient care with the laser, as appropriate.

Nursing roles and lasers

The role of the nurse in laser treatment may vary with clinical setting and with state of licensure. It is the nurse's responsibility to ensure he or she is knowledgeable of his or her own scope of practice and the requirements of the facility and the state board of nursing. The nurse must also ensure that any competencies are maintained and that he or she stays abreast of the latest technology and treatments available using evidence-based information in practice.

Many nurses have taken great satisfaction in providing care for their patients that includes application of laser therapy, teaching, and wound care for treated patients, all in one visit. The patient can benefit from the nurse's full potential.

Preoperative care of the laser patient

When selecting a patient for laser treatment, it is essential that the patient have realistic goals and expectation of outcomes. The patient must understand all the risks, benefits, and alternatives, and all the patient's questions must be answered before a treatment. The appropriate laser for the patient must be selected, and any contraindications must be determined. In the author's clinic, pregnancy is a contraindication, although no specific studies have been performed.

Patients should complete the full informed consent process with each treatment. The patient should understand that with all laser or light-source treatments, the risks include, but are not limited to, bruising, swelling, hypopigmentation, hyperpigmentation, recurrence, incomplete treatment, temporary improvement, infection, and scar. Patients should be encouraged to ask as many questions as they wish and should express verbally and in writing that they agree to have the procedure performed.

Potential contraindications include isotretinoin intake within the past 1 or 2 years, a history of hypertrophic scarring or keloids, recent therapies such as chemical peeling, recent sun exposure, a history of pigmentary changes related to laser therapy, and unrealistic expectations. Patients who have darker skin types should be warned of possible pigmentary changes following laser treatment. These pigmentary changes are usually transient and, in the author's experience, resolve within 1 to 6 months. Patients with a suntan usually are not treated, because the tan may prevent uptake of energy to the target vessels in the dermis and increase absorption in the epidermal melanin, thus increasing the risk of pigmentary changes. Pre- and postoperative photographs can important for documenting improvement. Patients often do not realize the extent of improvement until they compare before and after photographs.

The nurse should ensure that the patient is as comfortable as possible during the laser procedure. A patient's pain tolerance is important when considering methods of pain control during the procedure. Most patients experience only a very brief stinging sensation with each pulse, similar to the snap of a rubber band, which often is well tolerated without anesthesia. Repeated pulses, however, may begin to cause pain for the patient. The use of topical anesthesia, such as a 4% lidocaine cream applied thickly 1 hour before the laser treatment and with or without occlusion, may reduce discomfort.

In some cases the patient will require local infiltration and nerve blocks using 1% to 2% lidocaine with epinephrine 1:100,000. Epinephrine is a vasoconstrictor and may reduce blood flow to some vascular lesions. It should be determined whether epinephrine might affect the efficacy of a treatment and perhaps should be withheld. Patients who are anxious or children who are unable to maintain positioning during a treatment may require oral or intravenous sedation or general anesthesia. The goal is for the nurse and the patient is to be prepared; the patient's comfort should be considered throughout laser treatment.

Postoperative care of the laser patient

A patient who has received any laser treatment should be informed fully about the recovery process. This information should be provided well before the treatment is administered. Laser-treated skin responds differently depending on the laser used, the skin type, and the target entity. Immediately after treatment, most patients experience a burning sensation that may last only a few minutes or may last several hours. If the face or a large area was treated, significant swelling may develop, especially around the mouth and eyes. Patients who have vascular anomalies treated with the PDL develop discolorations the size of a laser spot, resembling a bruise, at the treatment site; these discolorations last 7 to 14 days. It is helpful to prepare prospective patients by showing a photograph of what to expect. It often is difficult to describe the appearance immediately after treatment, and patients often are shocked. Patients treated with other vascular lasers experience some pink or red discoloration of the skin at or around the treatment site and also may develop some crusting, which often fades in 1 to 3 days. General principles of care are similar for all treated skin. Box 1 contains the recommendations made by the author's clinic.

Box 1. General care for laser-treated skin

1. Do not rub, scratch or put pressure on the laser-treated area for 48 hours.
2. The treatment areas may become swollen, especially around the eyes.
3. Apply ice 10 minutes every hour for the first day and then intermittently if swelling persists.
4. You may bathe or shower. A gentle soap is recommended. You may use baby shampoo to cleanse around the eye area to avoid irritation to the eye.
5. If the skin fully intact, make-up can be worn.
6. You must be very cautious about exposure to the sun for the next 6 weeks and use sunscreen with a sun protection factor of 30 or higher. A hat with full coverage is recommended if you anticipate that you will be exposed to the sun for prolonged periods of time. (It is recommended that a patient who has been treated with amino levulinic acid and laser treatment [a photodynamic therapy that greatly increases sun sensitivity] have no exposure to the sun for at least 48 hours).
7. It can take up to 6 weeks for all to show a response at the treatment site, and most lesions take multiple sessions.
8. Avoid aspirin or ibuprofen products, which may increase the risk of bruising, for 5 days before treatment.

In addition to general care, patients should be informed of postoperative considerations relevant to their specific treatment. Box 2 shows the guidelines used in the author's clinical setting.

Laser complications

As with any procedure in dermatology, there are risks of complications. With lasers the most likely complications are bruising, infection, scar, incomplete treatment, recurrence, hyperpigmentation, hypopigmentation, and discomfort. The best prevention of any complication, of course, is preparation. The nurse should be trained adequately and obtain current knowledge about normal skin response, appropriate treatment modalities for skin conditions, and laser and energy requirements. This knowledge comes with time and experience and never should be rushed. Any provider performing laser treatments for patients should go through a complete orientation process, receive training sessions as laser technology advances, and keep abreast of new literature in the field of laser therapy. Appreciating the nuances of skin types and laser types takes time and patience. No expert

Box 2. Postoperative considerations for specific laser treatments

Blood vessels and redness
1. The treated area will be red and flushed for up to 24 hours, with some swelling, especially around the eyes and mouth.
2. Some of the blood vessels may become only slightly bruised. This bruising should resolve in 4 to 7 days.
3. In cases such as port-wine stains and flushing, the treatment intentionally causes intense bruising to achieve optimal results. The bruising will last 7 to 14 days.
4. Usually more than one treatment is needed to clear blood vessels.

Brown spots/pigmentation
1. When treated with the IPL or ruby laser, the spots or pigmented area will turn darker, and the skin will gradually slough over the next 5 to 7 days and then peel off. Do not pick at the treated areas.
2. Treatment with the pigment laser cause some superficial crusting. Apply petrolatum ointment for the first 2 to 3 days until crusting subsides. The spots will become darker and peel off over 5 to 7 days.
3. Usually more than one treatment is needed to clear the brown spots.

Tattoos
1. Apply petrolatum ointment to the treated site twice daily for 1 week.
2. If necessary, cover the site with a nonstick dressing to avoid rubbing by clothing.
3. There may be blistering and superficial crusting. Do not pick at the spots.
4. The pigment will have been shattered by the laser light and will be absorbed by your body over the next 4 to 6 weeks. Multiple treatments will be necessary.
5. Please notify your provider if you notice any itching near the site or a rash develops.

Hair removal
1. You may notice some swelling and redness around the hair follicle for 1 to 2 days after treatment.
2. It is normal for the treated hair to grow after the treatment.
3. Over the course of treatment, the number and the caliber of the hairs will diminish.
4. Expect at least five to six treatment sessions.

laser nurse developed his or her skills without extensive training and expo-sure to multiple patient types.

Alternatively, complications should be expected . Most complications are self-limiting and generally resolve without other sequelae. Lasting effects include persistent redness, scar, and recurrence. In the case of persistent red-ness, other laser treatment may reduce this side effect. In some cases, time is the only cure. In still others, there may be no treatment available.

In the case of a hypertrophic scar, which is an uncommon occurrence, improvement of bulky, red scars may be achieved with PDL to reduce some bulk and, especially, the redness. In some cases, adjuvant steroid injec-tion into the scar will result in faster resolution. Overall, the patient should understand that a scar is permanent and never will disappear completely.

For recurrence, re-treatment is required. The patient should understand before treatment that the estimated number of treatments is only that, an estimate. Whether the estimate is 1 or 10, the number of required treatments cannot always be predicted. The patient always should understand that re-treatment may be required.

For transient side effects and complications, patients should received education and reassurance. Pigment changes generally resolve more quickly with the avoidance of sun and, in some instances, with the use of a bleaching cream. Bruising and swelling are quite common; therefore all patients should anticipate both side effects. Infection is a risk in laser-treated areas where the skin breaks down and is more likely to occur with the ruby laser and tattoo treatments. Patients may require antibiotics, and, in some cases in which an aggressive treatment is performed, the patient may receive prophylactic oral antibiotics or antibiotic ointment for wound care.

Regardless of the type of side effect or complication, a patient needs to be reassured that everything possible will be done to help achieve the best possible outcome. The patient should be followed until resolution or until no further improvement is obtainable. The nurse has a vital role in provid-ing compassion and understanding in any event that causes a patient distress or concern. A patient's anxiety never should be dismissed or disregarded. A nurse can provide the reassurance that a patient needs to feel hopeful that the best care will be provided through this difficult time.

Summary

Nurses have become an essential part of patient care in laser therapy. In dermatology, the potential for helping patients achieve excellent results for individual skin needs is exponential when combined with appropriate tech-nology, evidence-based care, and a competent, conscientious nurse. Advances in laser technology are ongoing, and it is the responsibility of the laser nurse to provide the patient with the most current regimen of care, combined with the valuable role of a caring nurse.

References

[1] Alora MB, Dover JS, Arndt KA. Lasers for vascular lesions. Dermatol Nurs 1999;11: 97–102, 105–7.

[2] Amin SP, Goldberg DJ. Clinical comparison of four hair removal lasers and light sources. J Cosmet Laser Ther 2006;8:65–8.

[3] Flateau D. 2007 How lasers work. LFI International. Available at: http://www. lfiinternational.com/abcs.asp. Accessed June 13, 2007.

[4] Burstein FD, Williams KJ, Schwentker AR, et al. Intralesional laser therapy treatment for hemangiomas: technical evolution. J Craniofac Surg 2006;17:756–60.

[5] Greppi I. Diode laser hair removal of the black patient. Lasers Surg Med 2001;28:150–5.

[6] Kopera D. Q-switched ruby laser in cosmetic dermatology. Proc Paper Laser Appl in Med and Dentist 1996;8–15.

[7] Lanigan SW. Incidence of side effects after laser hair removal. J Am Acad Dermatol 2003;49: 882–6.

[8] Sundine MJ, Wirth GA. Hemangiomas, an overview. Clin Pediatr 2007;46:206–21.

[9] Laser hazards. OSHA technical manual. [Section 3: chapter 6]. Available at: http://www. osha.gov/dts/osta/otm/otm_iii/otm_iii_6.html#3. Accessed June 1, 2007.

[10] Willey A, Torrontegui J, Azpiazu J, et al. Hair stimulation following laser and intense pulsed light photo-epilation: review of 543 cases and ways to manage it. Lasers Surg Med 2007;39: 297–301.

[11] Marcus J, Goldberg DJ. Lasers in dermatology: a nursing perspective. J Dermatol Nurs 1996;8:181–7, 191–5, 204.

[12] Parlette EC, Groff WF, Kinshells MJ, et al. Optimal pulse durations for the treatment of leg telangiectasias with a neodymium YAG laser. Lasers Surg Med 2006;38:98–105.

NURSING
CLINICS
OF NORTH AMERICA

Nurs Clin N Am 42 (2007) 407–419

Atopic Dermatitis

Susan Tofte, RN, MS, FNP-C

Department of Dermatology, Oregon Health & Science University,
3303 SW Bond Avenue, Mail Code CH16D, Portland, OR 97239, USA

Atopic dermatitis (AD) is a chronic inflammatory skin disease characterized by intense pruritus and frequent relapsing courses. It occurs mostly in patients who have a personal or family history of other atopic conditions, such as asthma or allergic rhinitis. The prevalence of AD is high, particularly in children, with rapidly increasing numbers in the past few decades. The chronicity of this disease, along with its relapsing nature, presents treatment and management challenges for clinicians and frustration for patients and their families.

Terminology

The terms *atopic dermatitis* and *atopic eczema* are used interchangeably [1]. They are often referred to as part of a triad, or more specifically, the *atopic triad*. The combination of AD, asthma, and allergic rhinitis create the atopic triad seen in approximately 80% of people affected with AD and are useful to help confirm the diagnosis of AD. The word *eczema* is derived from a Greek word meaning to effervesce or literally to "boil over." The general term *eczema* is often used alone to describe itchy skin rashes and is inaccurately used synonymously with atopic dermatitis or atopic eczema. It is actually a generic term used to describe many different types of inflammatory conditions, including nummular eczema, AD, and contact (allergic and irritant) dermatitis, all of which are characteristically erythematous, pruritic, and frequently papulovesicular. Patients who have AD are often said to have a history of atopy, referring to the genetic predisposition for exaggerated skin and mucosal reactivity (pruritus, bronchospasm, rhinorrhea, and inflammation).

E-mail address: toftes@ohsu.edu

0029-6465/07/$ - see front matter © 2007 Elsevier Inc. All rights reserved.
doi:10.1016/j.cnur.2007.06.002   *nursing.theclinics.com*

Diagnosing

Atopic dermatitis is primarily a childhood disease. In the United States, approximately 17% of children and 1% to 3% of adults are affected [2]. Most children are diagnosed early, with more than 60% presenting in infancy before the first year of life and 90% within the first 5 years [3]. Age of onset is an important diagnostic feature; late onset suggests the need to at least consider the possibility of another diagnostic entity, such as contact dermatitis or cutaneous lymphoma, especially for cases unresponsive to therapy. In infancy, the disease will usually present on the face and extensor flexors. In older children and adults it is more likely to involve flexural areas (antecubital and popliteal fossae) and the trunk, although it can appear on the scalp, face, neck, and other parts of the body. Of children diagnosed in early years, an estimated 40% outgrow it before school age, but many others will have disease that persists well into the teen years and into adulthood.

Diagnosing AD correctly is important to treat patients appropriately. Criteria developed decades ago by Hanifin and Rajka [4] remain the standard for diagnosing AD. These criteria were recently modified by the American Academy of Dermatology (AAD) consensus conference to be more inclusive for infants and various ethnicities, and are listed in Box 1 [4,5].

The original criteria list several key diagnostic features and minor features that help diagnose AD. Essential criteria include the presence of itch and typical morphology and distribution patterns; facial, neck, and extensor involvement in infants and young children; and current or prior flexural involvement in older children and adults, sparing groin and axillae at any age. Other modifiers are not always present, but approximately 80% of patients will show at least some of these features. Box 2 lists the suggested universal criteria for diagnosing AD.

The causes of AD are not fully understood, but dysregulation of the immune system as evidenced in the imbalance of T-helper cells, Th1 and Th2 responses, and poor function of the skin barrier are significant elements in the origin of the disease [1,6]. A combination of genetic and environmental factors is likely to have a role in disease development and exacerbations.

The recent groundbreaking report of Iq21 filaggrin mutations in ichthyosis vulgaris and the strong association with AD and asthma [7] highlights the importance of assessing patients and family members not only for atopic features but also for the ichthyosis triad, including keratosis pilaris and hyperlinear palms. Early treatment of xerosis may prevent later problems with allergic disease [6–8] and epidermal barrier defects [6,9].

Laboratory testing

No laboratory markers exist for AD. Elevated IgE levels, often seen in patients who have AD and once considered a prerequisite for diagnosing AD, are now considered nonspecific and seldom necessary for diagnosis

Box 1. Guidelines for the diagnosis of atopic dermatitis

Must have three or more basic features
    Pruritus
    Typical morphology and distribution
        Flexural lichenification or linearity in adults
        Facial and extensor involvement in infants and children
    Chronic or chronically relapsing dermatitis
    Personal or family history of atopy (eg, asthma, allergic
        rhinitis, atopic dermatitis)
Plus three or more minor features
    Xerosis
    Ichthyosis/palmar hyperlinearity/keratosis pilaris
    Immediate (type I) skin test reactivity
    Elevated serum IgE
    Early age of onset
    Tendency toward cutaneous infections (especially
        Staphylococcus aureus and herpes simplex) and impaired
        cell-mediated immunity
    Tendency toward nonspecific hand or foot dermatitis
    Nipple eczema
    Cheilitis
    Recurrent conjunctivitis
    Dennie-Morgan infraorbital fold
    Keratoconus
    Anterior subcapsular cataracts
    Orbital darkening
    Facial pallor/facial erythema
    Pityriasis alba
    Anterior neck folds
    Itch when sweating
    Intolerance to wool and lipid solvents
    Perifollicular accentuation
    Food intolerance
    Course influenced by environmental/emotional factors
    White dermographism/delayed blanch

From Hanifin JM, Rajka G. Diagnostic features of atopic dermatitis. Acta Derm Venereol (Stockh) 1980;92(Suppl):44–7.

or treatment. Skin prick tests or radioallergosorbent tests (RASTs) may be useful when patients who have AD present with accompanying respiratory conditions and for determining food allergies, especially in infants and children [4].

Box 2. Suggested universal criteria for atopic dermatitis

Essential features that must be present and, if complete, are
   sufficient for diagnosis
   Pruritus
   Eczematous changes that are acute, subacute, or chronic
      Typical and age-specific patterns
         Facial, neck, and extensor involvement in infants and
            children
         Current or prior flexural lesions in adults/any age
         Sparing of groin and axillary regions
      Chronic or relapsing course
Important features that are seen in most cases, adding support
   to the diagnosis
   Early age at onset
   Atopy (IgE reactivity)
   Xerosis
Associated features
   Clinical associations help suggest the diagnosis of AD but are
      too nonspecific to be used to define or detect AD for
      research and epidemiologic studies
   Keratosis pilaris/ichthyosis/palmar hyperlinearity
   Atypical vascular responses
   Perifollicular accentuation/lichenification/prurigo
   Ocular/periorbital changes
   Perioral/periauricular lesions
Exclusions
   Firm diagnosis of AD depends on excluding conditions, such
      as scabies, allergic contact dermatitis, seborrheic
      dermatitis, cutaneous lymphoma, ichthyoses, psoriasis, and
      other primary disease entities

Adapted from Eichenfield LF, Hanifin JM, Luger TA, et al. Consensus conference on pediatric atopic dermatitis. J Am Acad Dermatol 2003;49:1088–95; with permission.

Treatment and management

The most effective management regimen for AD comes from a confident and well-reasoned approach. A combined approach involving experienced clinicians and dedicated nurses optimizes the patient education process and ensures greater patient compliance and more positive outcomes. Controlling a severe relapsing disease often requires a combination of therapies, education, and creativity.

Bathing/moisturizing

The simplest and most basic, although most misunderstood, treatment for AD is proper bathing and moisturizing. Errors in bathing and moisturizing are the most common cause of persistent AD. Patients are often confused by two true but opposing facts: (1) bathing dries the skin—TRUE: water left to evaporate off the skin causes the stratum corneum (outer layer of skin) to contract, leading to cracks and fissures and ultimately impairing the epidermal barrier, and (2) bathing hydrates the skin—ALSO TRUE, if adequate moisturizer is applied to damp/wet skin within 3 minutes of exiting the water, thereby trapping moisture in the skin and allowing the stratum corneum to retain flexibility and remain soft. In normal skin, the stratum corneum forms an outside barrier that protects skin cells from toxins and irritants. The compromised barrier seen in patients who have AD leads to increased and continual water loss, with eventual overall xerosis and often microscopic cracks in the skin, providing a portal of entry for damaging and infectious toxins. Daily bathing is preferred over infrequent baths, especially for those who have flares that are difficult to control. Cleansing and hydrating allow for enhanced penetration of topical corticosteroids and moisturizers, and bathing is generally a relaxing and enjoyable time for children and adults. A 20-minute warm soaking tub bath is preferable, although even a brief shower provides some hydrating benefit. Allowing children to negotiate swim time for bath time gives them some control over their disease, is fun, and is a reasonable bath substitute, providing the same hydration that a soaking bath provides. The choice of soap is less important than actual soaking, but if patients are concerned, unscented Dove, Olay Sensitive Skin, and Cetaphil liquid cleanser or bar soap are gentle and generally less irritating. If patients are concerned about soap causing increased dryness, clinicians can suggest limiting its use to cleansing the axillae, groin, and toe web spaces. Occasionally adding salt to the bath water (1 cup per full tub of water) helps make the water more like the body's natural physiologic fluids and may ease the stinging and discomfort sometimes associated with soaking when the skin is excoriated or weeping, or has open sores.

Education about proper moisturizing is as important as education about proper bathing. The "3 minute rule" (ie, applying emollient or topical steroid within 3 minutes of getting out of the water) is a helpful instruction for patients and helps ensure adequate and proper moisturization. Many good lubricating and well-tolerated nonfragranced moisturizers are available, such as Cetaphil cream, Vanicream, Aveeno cream, Eucerin, or plain petrolatum. Clinicians should emphasize to patients that lotions, because of their high water and alcohol content, will actually remove moisture from the skin, thereby increasing dryness and scaling, whereas cream or ointment-based emollients add softness and pliability to the skin and are always preferred. Patients should be instructed to choose moisturizers that must be scooped from a jar or squeezed from a tube rather than ones found in pump or pour bottles. Bath oils may be added to bath water if patients prefer, but should never be considered a substitute for applying a good moisturizing cream or ointment after bathing.

Skin "barrier" therapies

In addition to creams and ointments, a recently approved class of mechanical products termed *hydrogels* (Atopiclair, MimyX, and Epiceram) may provide benefits for some patients.

Topical steroids

Topical steroids have been the mainstay for treating AD for many decades; however, many clinicians have an approach/avoidance conflict regarding their safety and efficacy, and patients and their families have fears about their use. A study by Charman and colleagues [10] found that 72.5% of patients or guardians had concerns about using topical steroids that interfered with their ability to maintain control of the disease. Patients prescribed multiple-strength therapies (weaker concentration for face, medium strength for body, and stronger for hands and feet) often experience confusion about how and where to use medications and fear about using them incorrectly, leading to noncompliance. When a class VII steroid is prescribed as solo therapy, patients often become discouraged when they see little response and give up completely, returning to the clinic frustrated and flaring or ending up in the emergency department for an out-of-control flare. This visit may result in patients being treated by inexperienced, unaware, nondermatologic physicians who, out of desperation, give oral and injectable steroids as a quick fix to treat patients quickly and move them out of the acute care and emergency settings. Short-term use of a mid-strength topical steroid (eg, triamcinolone, mometasone, fluticasone) is preferable to prolonged but less-effective use of a lower-potency steroid (eg, hydrocortisone) and safer than oral or intramuscular steroids. When used appropriately, they will calm an acute flare within a few applications.

As important as choosing the correct medication is knowing how much and where to apply it. Medications should be applied immediately after a soaking bath twice daily for 3 to 7 days to achieve flare control. Twice weekly use of this regimen can be continued safely for long-term maintenance after the flare is controlled. Steroids with an ointment base are always preferred over one with a cream base because of their improved lubricating effect and are less likely to cause irritation from preservative additives that are necessary in creams. Although short-term controlled use of a mid-strength steroid is safe and effective, clinicians must emphasize that daily long-term use can lead to thinning of the skin and eventual steroid atrophy.

In addition to prescribing the correct strength of steroid, adequate quantities must be prescribed—enough to treat all affected areas twice daily for at least 7 days. Frequently clinicians provide too little medication (especially for adults who have widespread disease) and therefore patients apply too little medication to try to make it last and treat only the worst lesions, ignoring the rest of their skin. Subsequently, they often return to the clinic for more medication, frustrated and flaring. Although steroids are considered first-line therapy for AD, the chronicity of this disease often requires an alternative or combination approach, adding nonsteroidal treatment modalities to the treatment plan. Topical immunomodulators or calcineurin inhibitors (eg, Elidel cream, Protopic ointment) have been available for the past several years and are approved for use in children as young as 2 years. Using a mid-strength steroid for several days to control acute flares, inflammation, and itch and then introducing a topical immunomodulator for maintenance is a reasonable and effective approach. This regimen often prevents the typical cutaneous side effects (eg, burning, increased itching, stinging) known to occur when topical immunomodulators are applied to inflamed or broken skin.

Topical immunomodulators

The newest class of medications approved for AD are the topical immunomodulators. Protopic (tacrolimus) comes in two strengths, 0.1% and 0.03%, and received approval from the U.S. Food and Drug Administration in 2001. The lower concentration (0.03%) is approved for children aged 2 to 15 years, and the higher concentration (0.1%) for adults and children older than 15 years. Elidel (pimecrolimus) cream received approval a year after Protopic and is approved for children aged 2 years and older who have mild to moderate AD. The most common side effects of the topical immunomodulators are cutaneous side effects, including burning, stinging, and itching. Patients must be warned about potential side effects so they are not alarmed when they occur. Patients who have not been adequately informed about side effects are likely to discontinue use after a few applications, because they are concerned that their disease is worsening or they are experiencing an unexpected side effect, losing the benefit of the drug. To maximize compliance, clinicians should emphasize that side effects usually subside within a few days. Clinicians must also emphasize that Elidel and Protopic can be used safely on the face, neck, and groin and other thin-skinned areas where application of steroids are generally avoided.

Antihistamines

Sedating antihistamines help provide a more restful sleep by preventing constant scratching during the night. Over-the-counter diphenhydramine at recommended doses or sedating prescription antihistamines, such as hydroxyzine or doxepin (generally used in doses of 25–75 mg for hydroxyzine and 10–30 mg for doxepin), can be used for this purpose. Although nonsedating antihistamines (eg, loratadine, fexofenadine hydrochloride, cetirizine) help reduce respiratory and nasal symptoms of seasonal or environmental allergies, little evidence supports their use during the daytime to reduce itching [11].

Systemic treatment

Severe or recalcitrant AD is disruptive and can be disabling. For these patients, systemic treatments may be considered. Frequent use of oral or intramuscular corticosteroids present safety issues but can be used for brief infrequent intervals to control acute flares. Taking prednisone in doses of 30 to 40 mg twice daily for 2 days and then reducing the dose by half every 2 days for a total of 6 days is a safe and effective approach for most patients who have severe AD. Instructing patients to begin adding topical steroids toward the end of the taper is important. Because AD is a chronic disease, using systemic steroids for other than brief occasional courses carries the liability of demands for prolonging this high-risk therapy; tachyphylaxis occurs and discontinuance always leads to rebound flaring. Patients should be aware of the many life-altering side effects of chronic use of systemic steroids, such as cataracts, glaucoma, and osteoporosis.

Other systemic immunosuppressants may also be used to manage the most severe, recalcitrant, and difficult-to-control conditions. These therapies include cyclosporin, azathioprine, mycophenolate mofetil, methotrexate, phototherapy, and interferon gamma, but should only be considered when all other therapies have failed to achieve remission and should only be considered when patients can be closely supervised by an experienced clinician.

Cyclosporin A is a highly effective immunosuppressant for patients who have the most severe AD [12]. It is prescribed in single daily doses of 5 mg/kg and usually provides prompt relief of itching and reduction of inflammation within the first 2 to 5 days. In rare cases when no response occurs within this period, the dose may be cautiously increased to 7 mg/kg until remission is achieved. Cyclosporin is then slowly tapered, usually to approximately 3 mg/kg. Patients should always be advised that treatment with cyclosporin is limited to 3 to 6 months because of possible side effects, which can include but are not limited to hypertension, reduced renal function (usually reversible), and interstitial fibrosis. A well-planned approach most often involves beginning to taper cyclosporin within 1 month of initiation of therapy and simultaneously starting a combination ultraviolet light therapy (UVA/UVB). This approach allows for continued clearing while cyclosporin is gradually discontinued. Because of the potential problem with hypertension, blood pressures should be checked weekly and chemistry panels performed biweekly.

Nifedipine, a calcium-channel blocker, is used to control moderate increases in blood pressure. Although it is a potent systemic immunomodulator, cyclosporin can even be used safely in children who have severe resistant disease, and is increasingly used by pediatric dermatologists. Aza-thioprine is an immunosuppressant drug that is often slow in onset and, al-though significantly less effective than cyclosporine, can be considered. Azathioprine is characterized by a high rate of hepatic and other side effects [13]. A trial of therapy in adults might be considered in doses of 100 to 200 mg daily for 1 month.

Interferon gamma is a biologic response modifier that is effective in most patients who have severe AD and those whose condition is not controlled with cyclosporin. The disadvantage of this therapy is the exceedingly high cost and the route of administration (subcutaneous injection). Flu-like ef-fects often seen with this therapy can be reduced or eliminated through dos-ing before bedtime or dosing in combination with acetaminophen. Patients tend to become more tolerant of the side effects with continued use [14].

Methotrexate, often used to treat psoriasis, can be effective for some pa-tients who have AD. Liver toxicity is always a concern but, when used in low doses of 2.5 mg daily 4 days per week (increasing to 5 days per week if needed) and with vigilant monitoring of liver function tests, it provides a safe and sometimes effective alternative therapy for patients whose condi-tion does not respond to other treatments.

Mycophenolate mofetil is an immunosuppressive agent that has been used for several years to treat severe AD and can be helpful for some pa-tients. Dosing is usually initiated at 1500 mg/d in adults, but some patients require doses twice as high to induce remission. Biologics, now used exten-sively to treat psoriasis, are possible treatment considerations for AD.

An open study of infliximab performed in Europe found few positive effects on dermatitis. A recent 3-month pilot study of efalizumab in 10 pa-tients who had severe AD noted definite improvement in most patients in the first 4 to 8 weeks of therapy, but these positive effects dissipated for most patients during the later stages of the study [15]. Generally few adverse effects were noted, aside from one patient who developed progressive throm-bocytopenia that continued after the drug was discontinued and who re-quired systemic corticosteroid therapy until the problem eventually resolved after 6 months off the drug.

Inpatient hospitalization can be considered for patients whose condition fails to respond to all other forms of therapy and who have adequate health benefits to cover the cost of services. Hospitalization helps facilitate clearing of skin inflammation to allow for patch testing and prick testing, and en-ables clinicians to control food avoidance and challenge. For many patients who have severe conditions, no other way exists to prepare them for testing, because this cannot occur when the patient is taking immunosuppressives or the skin is widely inflamed. Even severe inflammation subsides spontane-ously with minimal treatment when patients are hospitalized, and marked improvement in skin and reduction of itching is usually seen within 24 to 48 hours. Part of the hospitalization plan is to institute a "rare foods" diet of rice, lamb, turkey, and low-allergenicity fruits and vegetables after the patient is admitted, adding a new food group (eg, eggs, dairy products) challenge each day to reassure patients or parents against the suspicion of food allergy causation. Patch tests can usually be applied after 3 to 4 days in the hospital and patients can be discharged 48 hours after the first patch test reading. After discharge, patients continue the in-hospital routine for the next 4 to 7 days, and then begin to slowly taper topical corticosteroids and substitute for topical immunomodulators or ultraviolet therapy. Many patients whose condition was formerly recalcitrant have experienced response to this intervention and have continued with greater stability of their disease. A follow-up clinic visit can be scheduled 5 to 7 days later for delayed patch test reading and to affirm the stability of maintenance therapy.

Exacerbating factors

Patients should aware of external factors that contribute to or cause flares. Infections of all types can cause AD flares, but viral infections such as upper respiratory infections (URIs) are the most common cause in infants and children. Although little can be done for a URI, it helps for parents to recognize it as the likely cause of AD flares and to know that generally the flare settles down when the virus has run its course. Bacterial infections, usually caused by *Staphylococcus aureus*, also trigger flares in AD. Teaching parents and patients to recognize the classic pustules or "pus bumps" (usually occurring on the upper and lower extremities) when the impaired skin barrier gets infected, and then quickly starting oral antibiotics, help halt severe flares.

Although judicious use of antibiotics is important to avoid causing antibiotic resistance, short courses can be safe and effective. Dicloxacillin or a cephalosporin (500 mg, 2–3 times daily for 5 days) is usually adequate for treating superficial infections and alleviates the concern about developing resistance. Newer-generation antibiotics do not promote speedier resolution of infections caused by *S aureus*. However, with the growing numbers of community-acquired methicillin-resistant *S aureus* infections, obtaining a bacterial culture in the most recalcitrant cases is indicated. For those cases, using alternative antibiotics, such as clindamycin, doxycycline, tetracycline, or trimethoprim–sulfamethoxazole, given with or without rifampin, may be necessary [16]. For occasional patients who have chronic recurrent infections, tetracycline used for 1 month can be considered along with application of topical antibiotics to the nares, umbilicus, and perineum daily for a week, then once weekly for a month. Topical Polysporin and mupirocin work well and are good choices. Using bleach in the bath water for patients who have frequent skin infections may also be helpful (adding a half cup of bleach to a tub of water), and using an antibacterial soap for cleansing may help with decolonization. The impaired barrier of atopic skin is also susceptible to other types of skin infections, such as yeast, tinea, molluscum contagiosum, and herpes simplex virus (HSV). Each of these infections can cause prolonged flaring, and therefore parents and patients should be educated to observe for signs of these infections and to seek appropriate treatment.

In general, topical antivirals are ineffective at treating HSV, but a course of oral acyclovir, 400 mg taken thrice daily for 5 days, is effective and should be started at the first sign of a herpes outbreak. Localized dermatophyte infections are treated with topical antifungals, whereas extensive skin or nail involvement are best treated with an oral azole antifungal. Molluscum contagiosum, commonly seen in childhood, is often widespread in children who have AD because of its tendency to spread when excoriated. It can be treated in the office with liquid nitrogen therapy or topical cantharidin, but when left alone will often resolve on its own.

Allergy versus skin care

Patients and parents frequently raise the issue of allergies. Confusion often exists about the connections between AD and allergic disease. Food allergy questions are at the forefront of concerns, particularly with infants and young children. Clinicians must clarify with patients whether they are seeing eczema or actual IgE-mediated reactions (eg, hives, lip swelling, respiratory, gastrointestinal symptoms) and help them recognize that eczema continues even when foods, pets, and mites are avoided. Food allergy, urticaria, respiratory, and gastrointestinal symptoms are common in patents who have AD and may be caused by antigens penetrating the compromised skin barrier but do not cause eczema on the skin.

When allergy is emphasized as a cause of eczema, patients and parents wrongly assume that food elimination will help cure the disease. Nutrients essential for normal development can be wrongfully withheld from children who have AD in an attempt to control their skin disease, potentially resulting in impaired growth. Food allergy testing is a last resort and is best used only for the most severe, recalcitrant conditions. Testing is performed for the six most common allergens: egg, milk, peanut, soy, wheat, and seafood, and the results are used in the RAST assessment. It is always best to stress to the patient that prick testing and RAST results are 90% accurate when negative, but that only 20% of the positive tests are relevant for AD [16–18]. The authors have found that when patients and parents focus on good skin care (eg, bathing, moisturizing, appropriate use of topical medications) rather than on suspect allergens, they are more likely to maintain control of the disease and prevent flares.

Impact of atopic dermatitis on quality of life

Dealing with a chronic inflammatory disease places financial and emotional burdens on families but, with a confident well-planned approach using a dedicated and experienced team, effective management can be achieved.

When AD develops in childhood (for most before 5 years of age), it comes at a critical time of psychosocial development for most children [19]; a time when children are learning about friendships, interactions, and social feelings. Having a chronic itchy, red skin disease interferes with children's ability to create and nurture friendships within their peer groups. Family members are also affected when the disease interferes with meals, vacations, and daily life. Children who have AD often require much more parental assistance and time to apply medications and moisturizers. Studies have shown that parents are 50% more likely to miss work when they have a child who has AD. The direct and indirect loss of work time and income is significant for these families. Sleep deprivation is a significant issue for all parents of children who have AD, with itching/scratching the major reason for sleep loss. Often the entire family is affected by the disruptive itch/scratch cycle at night; school and work performances are affected when family members experience sleep deprivation. Although intellectually capable, children will have difficulty concentrating on school activities when they do not get enough sleep to allow for adequate concentration during the day. Studies show that children who have AD are more irritable, fussy, and clingy. Parents of children who have AD are less likely to seek employment outside the home and participate in outside activities. Caring for a child who has severe AD also puts considerable emotional stress on marriages and relationships.

AD impacts all aspects of family life and health and creates a substantial social burden. Meals, activities, and vacations must be planned around family members who have AD. Studies show that caring for a child who has moderate to severe AD has a greater impact on families than caring for one who has type 1 diabetes mellitus. The cost of care for patients who had AD in the United States between 1990 and 1991 exceeded $300 million. These numbers increase in proportion to the rising prevalence of this disease, impacting not only families but also health care providers. Health care systems are burdened by disproportionate numbers of AD cases presenting to emergency departments and urgent care clinics [20]. Overall quality of life can be significantly impacted by AD, particularly from sleep loss caused by itching, ultimately leading to poor school or work performance and productivity.

Summary

AD is a difficult disease to manage and takes a multidisciplinary approach to achieve success. The disease creates a considerable social impact and affects all family members. Effective management is time consuming for both patient and clinician and begins with patient and caregiver education, including the importance of proper skin care, recognition of infections, trigger factors for flares, and appropriate use of medications. Patients often find help and support from organizations, such as the National Eczema Association (info@nationaleczema.org).

References

[1] Simpson EL, Hanifin JM. Atopic dermatitis. J Am Acad Dermatol 2005;53(1):115–28.

[2] Laughter D, Istavan J, Tofte S, et al. The prevalence of atopic dermatitis in Oregon school children. J Am Acad Dermatol 2000;43:649–55.

[3] Kay J, Gawkrodger DJ, Mortimer MJ, et al. . The prevalence of childhood atopic eczema in a general population. J Am Acad Dermatol 1994;30:35–9.

[4] Hanifin JM, Rajka G. Diagnostic features of atopic dermatitis. Acta Derm Venereol (Stockh) 1980;92(Suppl):44–7.

[5] Eichenfield LF, Hanifin JM, Luger TA, et al. Consensus conference on pediatric atopic dermatitis. J Am Acad Dermatol 2003;49(6):1088–95.

[6] Hudson TJ. Skin barrier function and allergic risk. Nat Genet 2006;38(4):399–400.

[7] Palmer CAN, Irvine AD, Terron-Kwiatkowski AT, et al. Common loss-of-function variants of the epidermal barrier protein filaggrin are a major predisposing factor for atopic dermatitis. Nat Genet 2006;38(4):441–6.

[8] Hanifin JM. Atopic dermatitis. In: Moschella SL, Hurley HJ, editors. Dermatology. 3rd edition. Philadelphia: W.B. Saunders Company; 1992. p. 441–64.

[9] Irvine AD, McLean WHI. Breaking the (un)sound barrier: filaggrin is a major gene for atopic dermatitis. J Invest Dermatol 2006;126:1200–2.

[10] Chaman CR, Morris AD, Williams HC. Topical corticosteroid phobia in patients with atopic eczema. Br J Dermatol 2000;142(5):931–6.

[11] Hanifin JM, Cooper KD, Ho VC, et al. Guidelines of care for atopic dermatitis, developed in accordance with the American academy of dermatology (AAD/American Academy of Dermatology Association "Administrative Regulations for Evidence based Clinical Practice Guidelines." J Am Acad Dermatol 2004;50(3):391–404.

[12] Sowden JM, Berth-Jones J, Ross JS, et al. Double-blind, controlled crossover study of cyclosporine in adults with severe refractory atopic dermatitis. Lancet 1991;338:137–40.

[13] Meggitt SJ, Gray JC, Reynolds NJ. Azathioprine dosed by thiopurine methyltransferase activity for moderate-to-severe atopic eczema: a double-blind, randomized controlled trial. Lancet 2006;367(9513):839–46.

[14] Hanifin JM, Schneider LC, Leung DYM, et al. Recombinant interferon-gamma therapy for atopic dermatitis. J Am Acad Dermatol 1993;28:189–97.

[15] Takiguchi RH, Tofte SJ, Simpson BM, et al. Efalizumab for severe atopic dermatitis—a pilot study in adults. J Am Acad Dermatol 2007;56(2):222–7.

[16] Moran GJ, Krishnadasan A, Gorwitz RJ, et al. Methicillin-resistant S. aureus infections among patients in the emergency department. N Engl J Med 2006;355:666–74.

[17] Sampson HA, Albergo R. Comparison of results of skin tests, RAST, and double-blind placebo-controlled food challenges in atopic dermatitis. J Allergy Clin Immunol 1984;74:26–33.

[18] Rowlands D, Tofte SJ, Hanifin JM. Does food allergy cause atopic dermatitis? Food challenge testing to dissociate eczematous from immediate reactions. Dermatol Ther 2006; 19(2):97–103.

[19] Chamlin SL, Frieden IJ, Williams ML, et al. Effects of atopic dermatitis on young American children and their families. Pediatrics 2004;114(3):607–11.

[20] Lapidus CS, Schwarz DF, Honig PJ. Atopic dermatitis in children: who cares? Who pays? J Am Acad Dermatol 1993;28:699–703.

ELSEVIER
SAUNDERS

Nurs Clin N Am 42 (2007) 421–455

NURSING
CLINICS
OF NORTH AMERICA

Cutaneous T-Cell Lymphoma: Overview and Nursing Perspectives

Sue A. McCann, MSN, RN, DNC[a,b,*]

[a]Department of Dermatology, University of Pittsburgh Medical Center,
190 Lothrop Street, Suite 145 Lothrop Hall, Pittsburgh, PA 15213, USA
[b]Department of Nursing, University of Pittsburgh Medical Center,
Pittsburgh, PA 15213, USA

Cutaneous T-cell lymphoma (CTCL) represents a heterogeneous subset of non-Hodgkin lymphomas. CTCL is an umbrella term encompassing multiple lymphoma variants. The two most common entities subsumed within the CTCL nomenclature are mycosis fungoides (MF) and Sézary syndrome (SzS). MF was first described in the 1800s by Jean-Louis Alibert, whose patient had deforming tumors of the face that appeared as heaped-up, fungating lesions, hence the name mycosis fungoides.

Less common variants of the MF subcategory include folliculotropic MF, granulomatous slack skin, and pagetoid reticulosis. Other less common CTCLs include adult T-cell leukemia/lymphoma, lymphomatoid papulosis, primary cutaneous large-cell anaplastic lymphoma, primary cutaneous extranodal natural killer-like/T-cell lymphoma (nasal type), and primary subcutaneous panniculitis-like T-cell lymphoma [1].

CTCL is a systemic lymphoreticular disease with its primary lesions originating in the skin because of the skin-homing nature of specific T cells originally predetermined to provide immunologic surveillance in the skin. These T lymphocytes expand clonally and may progress to involve lymph nodes and viscera as well the skin [2,3].

In this article, the term "CTCL" is used to denote both MF and SzS. The "Nursing Notes" sections throughout the article are based on the author's 20 years of clinical experience in caring for patients living with CTCL. It has been a rich learning experience to provide nursing care to this group of patients and their families; some of that experience is shared here.

---

* Department of Dermatology 190 Lothrop Street, Suite 145 Lothrop Hall, Pittsburgh, PA 15213.

E-mail address: mccannsa@upmc.edu

Epidemiology

MF and SzS are the most common of the CTCLs with MF being the most prevalent. It is difficult to determine the actual prevalence of the disorder, since it is often indolent and chronic, lasting in many cases for decades. CTCL is most common in the later decades of life, beginning on average at the 5th or 6th decade, but any age group can be affected. The most recent U.S. study on incidence revealed a 2.9×10^{-6} increase per decade since 1973 with a current estimated incidence of 6.4 per million persons. It more commonly affects men with a 2:1 ratio over women and African Americans experience an increased incidence of 1.5:1 over Caucasians [4].

Etiology

The cause of CTCL remains unknown despite epidemiologic attempts to establish an infectious, environmental, or genetic link [5]. Some cases of multiple family members developing CTCL have been reported; however, there are no established genetic links [6]. Its pathology reflects a cancer of the immune system whereby the skin-homing T cells, preprogrammed to protect the skin, expand clonally, function in an activated state, and achieve clonal dominance [2]. This neoplastic, clonal expansion, generally of the CD4+ T-cell phenotype, ultimately produces the characteristic skin findings in MF and SzS: patches, plaques, erythroderma, and tumors.

Prognosis

Prognosis is good for patients who present with early-stage CTCL, with longevity approaching that of age-matched control groups and with relatively few reported disease-related deaths. In the advanced stages (IIB–IVB), however, the prognosis is less favorable. Disease-related deaths usually involve the overt failure of the immune system, leading to sepsis or other opportunistic infections [7].

Nursing notes

Patients frequently ruminate about the lack of an identified cause for CTCL. It is common for a patient to seek answers from multiple caregivers for the same question, "How did I get this?" Concerned that they may have done something to cause the CTCL, patients reflect on past employment and experiences, searching for a possible cause. Other patients worry that they will pass this disorder on to their children and even experience what they describe as nightmares about someone they love also developing the disease. Patients need health care professionals to provide multiple reassurances that the evidence to date in determining a cause for CTCL remains inconclusive and unknown. This information can be imparted to the patient through reassuring phrases such as, "You did nothing to cause this," "You can't pass this on to your family," and "No one can catch this from you."

The discussion surrounding prognosis may cause anxiety for patients. Even some patients who have stage IA disease worry a great deal about dying from the disease. This anxiety was evident in a recent survey on factors affecting quality of life, in which 80% of respondents reported worrying about dying [8]. Patients, especially those who have early-stage disease, need continual reinforcement that CTCL usually is a chronic disease and the prognosis is good for most patients. For patients who have advanced-stage disease, it is helpful to emphasize that new treatment modalities have become available recently, more clinical trials than ever before are open to CTCL patients, the longevity predictions in the literature most often indicate the natural history of the disease without treatment, and the prognostic statistics do not reflect accurately the effect new therapeutic modalities have on CTCL. It is important to remain honest but positive while emphasizing to the patient that he/she is not a statistic and that each experience is unique and personal.

Skin manifestations and symptoms

In the less common variants of MF, unique lesions are observed. Granulomatous slack skin presents as infiltrating lesions, primarily of the axillary/inguinal folds. Over time, the skin in these areas becomes atrophic and loses elasticity, and excessive skin folds are noted. Folliculotropic MF infiltrates hair follicles and produces localized alopecia. Pagetoid reticulosis is characterized by a localized keratotic or psoriasiform plaque that develops slowly and usually is found on a lower extremity [9]. In most patients who have classic MF, the rash or lesions are light pink to red; however, in some cases, depending on skin color or type of CTCL, the lesions may be purple in color, hypopigmented (white or lacking pigment), or hyperpigmented (brown-black), especially in dark skinned individuals. In the typical presentation, skin lesions are distributed in the bathing suit area (ie, trunk, buttocks, and sun-shielded areas of arms/legs), but they may be located on any body area [2]. The bathing suit area often is doubly protected by clothing throughout the lifespan and therefore is shielded more often from the effects of UV light (UVL), possibly predisposing this region to the early MF lesions.

There are four typical descriptions for skin changes in CTCL. The terms for these basic descriptions are patch, plaque, tumor, and erythroderma.

- In patients who have patch-type skin changes, a flat, discolored macule, most often pink to red in color, is observed (Fig. 1). When a patch is palpated, no discernable difference can be noted between normal and abnormal skin (ie, no induration is present, and the skin feels normal).

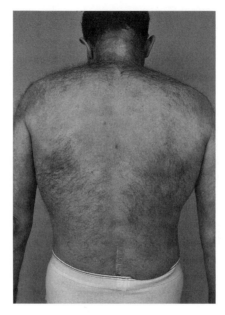

Fig. 1. Patch CTCL.

- A plaque is an elevated, discolored lesion, most often deep pink or red. With palpation, a distinct difference is evident relative to the thickness of the skin and the depth of the lesion when compared with unaffected skin (Figs. 2 and 3). Plaques may be thin or thick; the extent of induration depends on the amount of infiltration in the lesion.
- Tumor lesions are nodular and heaped-up with deep red to purple pigmentation. Tumor stage carries with it a worse prognosis because the cells in these lesions behave in a more aggressive, malignant manner, invading deeper tissue within the skin and subcutaneous tissue and resulting in vertical growth [2,10]. These tumors are often fragile, ulcerate easily, and become infected readily, causing pain and disability (Figs. 4 and 5).
- In erythrodermic CTCL, 80% or more of the patient's body surface area (BSA) is covered with reddened skin. The affected areas may be entirely patchlike in nature, or plaques and/or tumors may be admixed in the lesion morphology. Erythroderma also is seen in patients who have SzS. Some patients present with erythrodermic MF and lack nodal abnormalities or the leukemic T-cell expansion in the blood.

SzS is the leukemic variant of MF in which atypical lymphocytes with classic convoluted or cerebriform nuclei are found circulating in the periphery. The International Society of Cutaneous Lymphoma recently set forth guidelines for the identification and diagnosis of SzS. (Box 1) [11].

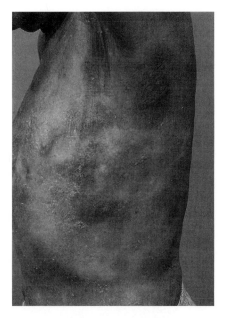

Fig. 2. Plaque CTCL.

In SzS, the extent of symptoms related to generalized erythema and scaling, referred to as "exfoliative erythroderma," can be overwhelming, debilitating, and devastating for patients. Because of the extensive scaling and skin shedding, iron, protein and electrolytes are lost through the skin, leading to electrolyte imbalance, anemia, hypoalbuminemia, and subsequent lower-extremity edema. Additionally, these patients have very poor body temperature control because of extensive vasodilation and shunting of blood to the skin. Even in warm temperatures, extra layers of clothing and/or blankets are necessary to maintain a comfortable body temperature. In

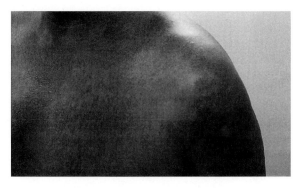

Fig. 3. Plaque CTCL in dark skin.

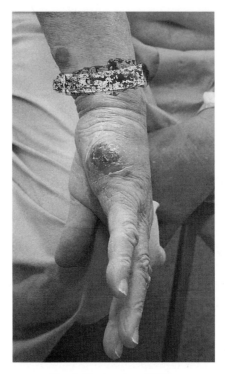

Fig. 4. Tumor-stage CTCL.

addition to erythroderma, other associated signs, most often found in erythroderma and SzS, include hyperkeratosis (thickened palmar/plantar skin) of
the palms and soles, fissuring of hands and feet, onycholysis and nail dystro-
phy, and alopecia (hair loss) in affected areas. In generalized erythroderma,
the patient may experience total body alopecia (Figs. 6–8). Another major
symptom for most patients is pruritus (itching) that may or may not be

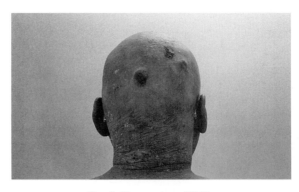

Fig. 5. Tumor-stage CTCL.

Box 1. Criteria for Sézary syndrome

Sézary count: absolute count of Sézary cells > 1000/mm^3
CD4/CD8 ratio > 10
Pan T-cell markers: CD4+/CD7−; CD4+/CD26− above normal
T-cell clone: positive by Southern blot or polymerase chain
    reaction analysis plus chromosomal abnormalities (deletions
    or translocations)

---

amenable to symptomatic treatment, including topical steroids, emollients, and a wide array of available oral antihistamines.

Nursing notes

Patients who have CTCL demonstrate a wide range of altered skin integrity and express a wide range of concerns related to it. These patients also are dealing with the associated symptoms of a chronic illness and a cancer diagnosis. Patients experience a variable amount of pruritus, at times intense and unremitting enough to produce severe emotional distress, depression, fatigue, and insomnia. Patients often complain that no matter what is prescribed for their itching, nothing really helps sufficiently.

Cold intolerance is especially problematic for patients who have erythroderma. It is common for patients to report having to wear a winter coat in the summer season. It is important to keep in mind that the "cold" erythrodermic patient may not always demonstrate a low-grade fever when infected, because the hypothermic-like state can mask the fever.

Skin pain and tenderness occur in some patients, especially those who have excoriations, ulcerations, fissuring, or infections of the skin lesions. Patients who have fissuring of the hands and feet suffer from pain, impaired dexterity, mobility, and ability to perform activities of daily living. The

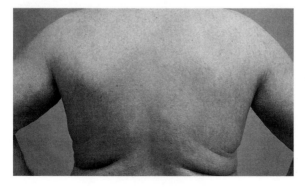

Fig. 6. Erythrodermic CTCL.

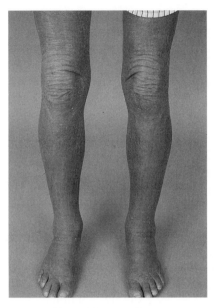

Fig. 7. Sézary syndrome.

patient may be unable to perform simple tasks such as closing buttons, opening cartons, or holding a pencil. It is difficult and painful to walk with fissured soles.

Patients have described living with CTCL as "being trapped inside my body" from which there is never any escape. Some patients also express significant embarrassment and anger related to having a visible skin disease and must deal with frequent stares because of visible skin lesions or the need for special clothing, protective eyewear, or cotton gloves for fissured hands. Other patients endure assumptions and admonitions from total

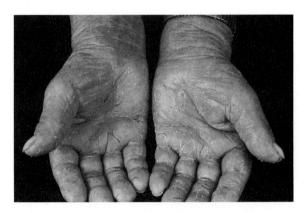

Fig. 8. Hyperkeratosis in Sézary syndrome.

strangers such as, "You should not get such a sun burn; it will give you cancer." Discussing these issues and developing a plan to deal with them (ie, cosmetic camouflage or general responses to insensitive comments) can be helpful.

Other common complaints include anxiety, fear, and depression related to having a chronic illness and being diagnosed as having cancer. As discussed previously, there is a fear, especially for those who have more advanced-stage disease or extensive skin involvement, of dying from the illness despite hearing (and reading) that they will most likely die from something else. Patients express a need to know about what dying with CTCL will be like. This question, of course, is difficult, if not impossible, to answer. Patients really need reassurance that the help and support to keep them comfortable and free of pain will be available if that time comes for them. Hospice services are invaluable at this stage.

Family dynamics often are strained, and patients report anger and frustration with family members who, they feel, do not take the disease seriously. Some patients feel the family member "just doesn't understand why I can't stop scratching or shedding all this dry skin that makes a mess out of the house." Patients may joke about having "blown up" or otherwise broken more than one vacuum cleaner because of daily use in cleaning up fallen, dead skin. Between the lines, these patients are reporting a burden experienced by themselves and their family that goes far beyond the sweeper.

Open discussions with trusted caregivers about problematic symptoms can help provide a framework the patient can use when dealing with symptom management and family stressors. For example, it sometimes is helpful to acknowledge with the patient and family that no matter what might be tried medically to alleviate pruritus, there are some cases where nothing seems to help. Alternative strategies to avoid the scratch–itch cycle then can be discussed (see the section "Nursing Role").

Diagnosis

The diagnosis of CTCL may be delayed by the difficulty in obtaining a diagnostic skin biopsy. It also is delayed when patients ignore asymptomatic, slow-growing, or changing lesions for months to years. It is common for patients to report the existence of the disease for some time before medical attention is sought or before a primary care physician refers the patient to a specialist. Often, multiple biopsies done over time (months to years) are required so that a histopathologic diagnosis can be made. CTCL is often called the "great mimicker" because the differential diagnosis of CTCL can be extensive. The most common misdiagnoses include psoriasis, allergic contact dermatitis, and eczema [3].

Staging is an important process in the management of CTCL patients. Management decisions usually are based on staging, and prognosis generally is correlated with stage at diagnosis, extent of tumor burden, and extracutaneous involvement throughout the course of the illness [12]. The prognosis for stage IA disease (involving < 10% BSA) is not different than for age-matched control groups, but the prognosis decreases with each subsequent stage. In contrast, the median overall survival from the time of diagnosis for stage IVA and IVB is only 1.5 to 2.5 years [13,14]. The diagnostic work-up to determine an accurate stage is divided into evaluations of skin tumor burden (T designation), nodal involvement (N designation), systemic metastasis (M designation), and blood involvement (B designation). The International Society for Cutaneous Lymphomas [11] has proposed using the extent of blood involvement as an additional staging criterion. The commonly used staging descriptions involving the TNM criteria are as follows:

- Stage IA: less than 10% BSA involved with patches or plaques (T1), no nodal abnormalities
- Stage IB: more than 10% BSA involved with patches or plaques (T2), no nodal abnormalities
- Stage IIA: any percentage of BSA involved with patches or plaques (T1–2) plus clinically abnormal lymph nodes
- Stage IIB: skin tumors (T3) with/without clinically abnormal lymph nodes
- Stage III: erythroderma (T4) with or without clinically abnormal lymph nodes (T4)
- Stage IVA: any extent of skin involvement (T1–4) but with positive lymph nodes
- Stage IVB: any extent of skin (T1–4) or nodal involvement but with metastasis to other organs

A patient's disease stage may change in response to therapy or from the natural history of the disease. Therefore, to reflect the disease history and progression accurately, patients' records may include the following staging data: stage at diagnosis, highest stage ever, and current stage. The stage at diagnosis often is considered the standard for determining overall prognosis. To achieve an accurate diagnosis and stage, multiple evaluations are required and involve clinical examinations, histopathology, hematology/chemistry, and radiographic imaging.

Clinical evaluations should be conducted by an experienced practitioner familiar with CTCL. This person usually is a specialized dermatologist or a hematologist/oncologist with expertise in cutaneous lymphomas. A complete history and physical examination, along with a full body examination, is needed to document the onset of skin rash or skin changes, accompanying symptoms, morphology, and distribution of lesions. A method of routinely documenting and recording skin changes is desirable so that progress or disease progression can be recorded and evaluated more objectively.

The physical examination also is important, because enlarged lymph nodes, liver, or spleen may be seen. In some cases, the experience of the clinician is the final determinant in establishing at least a provisional diagnosis, especially when skin biopsies remain nondiagnostic despite many repeated efforts. This experience is critical for the patient who requires initiation of appropriate therapy despite the lack of a firm diagnosis.

Skin biopsies provide the key to diagnosis because of the cutaneous nature of the disease. Tissue immunophenotyping aids greatly in establishing the diagnosis and specific cell type involved. As previously mentioned, repeated biopsies may be required to elicit a confirmed diagnosis. Lymph node biopsies are indicated for clinically enlarged lymph nodes. With fresh tissue and experienced laboratory analysis, flow cytometry and gene rearrangement also are useful tests to determine the ratio of CD4 to CD8 cells (an elevated ratio is a ratio of CD4 to CD8 cells > 4:1), the specific type of cellular involvement, and the presence of clonal lymphocytes (ie, CD4+ lymphocytes that lack expression of surface T-cell markers such as CD5, CD7, and CD26) [3,15].

Analysis of the blood is helpful on several levels. Although not specific for CTCL, routine hematology and chemistry evaluations are performed with specific interest in the complete blood cell count and peripheral blood smear to determine an elevated white blood cell count or the presence of atypical lymphocytes such as the characteristic cerebriform Sézary cells. Blood chemistry is useful to determine overall health with liver and kidney function along with lactate dehydrogenase, albumin, and uric acid. Peripheral blood flow cytometry and gene rearrangement studies (T-cell receptor beta chain) by Southern blot and polymerase chain reaction gamma chain help determine clonal blood involvement and phenotype, as described previously in the section on tissue diagnosis.

Diagnostic imaging with CT and/or positron-emission tomography/CT scans can rule out metastatic disease.

Lymph node biopsy should be performed in patients who have clinically abnormal lymph nodes and stage IIB disease or higher or as otherwise indicated by physical/diagnostic work-up.

Bone marrow biopsy should be considered in some patients, depending on staging and clinical presentation (ie, SzS). Routine bone marrow biopsy remains controversial.

Nursing notes

The delay in diagnosis experienced by some patients leads to a multitude of emotional hurdles that patients must work through to arrive at a place of acceptance related to their disease. Patients repeatedly discuss the unique scenario that delayed their diagnosis and express anger at physicians who were not able to "figure this out" or who "treated me for psoriasis for years." Patients even may blame themselves for ignoring disease symptoms for some time or for not being more insistent about seeing a specialist. They grieve over their perceived lost time and the lost opportunity of possibly attaining a remission; they may regard early diagnosis as offering potential cure. For these reasons, patients may become stuck in a phase of anger and denial related to the delayed diagnosis and initiation of the appropriate therapy. Again, it is important for patients to hear that their situation is common and that, even in the best hands, a microscopic diagnosis can take months and require repeated biopsies. Repeated emphasis on the current situation with initiation of appropriate therapy is helpful and provides the framework for the patient to move toward acceptance of the illness.

Treatment

A multidisciplinary approach often is required for patients who have more extensive skin involvement, generally greater than stage IA. For these patients, an interdisciplinary plan of care involving the dermatologist, oncologist, and radiation oncologist often improves outcomes and establishes a network of providers for multiple therapeutic pathways [16].

There are many therapeutic options for CTCL. This variety of options generally means there is no one or two therapies that work for most cases, most of the time, over an extended period of time. Available options may be subdivided into two major categories: those directed at the skin itself and those given systemically by mouth, intralesionally, subcutaneously, or intravenously. Within the past 10 to 20 years, a number of new therapies have emerged and have been approved by the Food and Drug Administration (FDA), and more are currently under study. CTCL is of interest in the study of potential new agents, because of its immunologic/oncologic pathology and the relative ease of determining the new agent's effectiveness through visual assessments of the skin. Because CTCL is designated as an orphan disease, the FDA review process may be given fast-track status, allowing new therapeutic options to become available more quickly.

Skin-directed therapy

Topical steroids

Throughout all stages of disease, topical steroids are a mainstay of therapy in helping relieve symptoms, decrease inflammation, suppress disease activity, and induce apoptosis. Typical regimens involve twice-daily applications to affected areas only (sparing the eye and/or face area, groin, and axillae). In an attempt to achieve clearing and for relatively short-term use in patch-stage disease, high-potency steroids (class I or II) may be tried as a first-line therapy. One pivotal study of 79 patients who had patch-stage disease with less than 10% BSA involvement (T1) demonstrated a remarkable 94% response rate. Sixty-three percent of these patients had a complete response, and 31% had a partial response. For patients who had patch lesions with greater than 10% BSA involvement (T2), there was an 82% response rate and a 25% complete response rate [17]. In a follow-up to that study of topical steroids, data including 200 patients were analyzed. The overall response rates were similar: 90% for T1 and 80% for T2 disease [18]. Topical steroids are used routinely as adjunctive therapy to alleviate symptoms and also to potentiate response to therapy. For long-term use, the use of the lowest potency possible to achieve the desired effects is recommended to avoid the side effects of long-term use (eg, striae, purpura, skin atrophy, and potential systemic effects from corticosteroid absorption, including adrenal corticoid hormone suppression) [10,14]. To minimize potential side effects, alternating treatment days with rest days is recommended. At the University of Pittsburgh Medical Center, several different rest/treatment patterns are used, including 2 weeks on followed by 1 week off therapy or therapy administered Monday through Friday with weekends off. During the off times, it is important to continue topical care with liberal emollient use.

For patients who have extensive erythroderma, steroid wet wraps can be very helpful in quickly reducing patient symptoms and restoring skin integrity more quickly. This rigorous regimen demands a great deal of effort from the patient and family. It is more easily accomplished during a bedtime ritual after the bath or shower. Following a bath and steroid application to the entire body surface (sparing axillae and groin), warmed, light-weight pajamas that have been wet with warm water and wrung out tightly should be applied, followed by thicker outerwear, such as a fleece jogging suit. Some patients find that warming the moistened pajamas briefly in the dryer before putting them on makes the process more comfortable. The patient then should go to bed for the evening with the goal of leaving the pajamas on for about 6 to 8 hours. Some relief of symptoms should be noted within several days. Initially, a Monday-through-Friday regimen with weekends off is desirable. Once the optimum effect is achieved, the regimen may be tapered slowly to prevent skin flare-up following abrupt withdrawal of steroids.

UV light

UVL phototherapy may be delivered in the clinic or with home light units, generally starting at three times per week, until clearing is achieved. The frequency of treatment then is tapered slowly to the minimum frequency that maintains the therapeutic effect. This therapeutic effect results from direct apoptosis and immunosuppression of activated T cells in the skin. Side effects vary somewhat depending on the type of light administered. In general, side effects increase in direct proportion to the cumulative dose of light and include hyperpigmentation, red or tan skin color, burns, early photoaging, and increased risk of skin cancers [19]. Administering light requires creativity and individualized planning, because areas of the body with natural shielding from UV light, such as the scalp, intertriginous areas, and the soles of the feet, may need alternative therapy or light specifically directed at the soles (with a hand/foot unit) or by a hand-held unit. Additionally, male genitalia must be shielded (male support garments work well) to prevent skin damage. The face or other frequently exposed skin areas may require additional shielding to prevent additional UV damage [10]. Patients who have a prior history of melanoma or basal cell or squamous cell skin cancers must use caution when undertaking this therapy and must be checked routinely and vigilantly for the development of new skin cancers. In the clinic, UVL therapy must be administered by specially trained staff and patient progress supervised routinely by the physician. Skin burns, sometimes severe, can occur from improper dosing of light, especially following a period when the patient did not receive the therapy routinely.

The physician may order different forms of UVL for the patient depending on the skin tumor burden, skin history and type, and proximity to a center where UVL is available. Psoralen plus UVA (PUVA) light therapy requires the patient to take an oral dose of the light-sensitizing agent psoralen about 90 minutes before the treatment. PUVA is used for the treatment of plaques and patches. UVA light has a longer wavelength and is able to penetrate deeper into the skin and therefore is more successful at treating plaques. Excellent response rates and long-lasting remissions have been seen with PUVA therapy [19]. Disadvantages of PUVA include the cost of psoralen and its associated side effects of nausea, headaches, and light-headedness. The nausea may be diminished by eating a consistent, nonfat meal just before taking the dose. Ginger products, such as ginger ale and ginger snaps, have been helpful to some patients routinely taking psoralen. Also, the light-sensitizing effects of the psoralen are systemic and require the patient to protect the skin and eyes for 24 hours following ingestion. Patients must limit sun exposure, using sunscreen with a minimum sun-protective factor of 15 and wearing wraparound UVL eye protection during this 24-hour interval. A less common but therapy-limiting side effect of PUVA is severe itching.

The shorter wavelength emitted by broadband UVB is more amenable to treating effectively only very thin plaques and patches because it does not penetrate as deeply as UVA light. No pills are required with UVB, and it may be administered by home units as patient ability and insurance coverage permit. More recently, narrowband UVB (NBUVB) has been used to treat CTCL. It may have efficacy similar to that of PUVA without the inherent problems of taking an oral photosensitizing agent [19] One study of eight patients who had patch-stage disease showed a 75% complete response rate with an average duration of 20 months [20]. Skin redness, photoaging, and itching are still potential side effects for UVB and NBUVB. UVB increases the risk for other skin cancers; less is known about the potential carcinogenic effects of NBUVB [14].

Nitrogen mustard

Nitrogen mustard (NM; mechlorethamine) is a topically applied chemotherapy administered in a water-based, gel, or petrolatum-based vehicle (the latter two are the more common methods). Although not approved by the FDA for topical use in CTCL, NM has been a mainstay of therapy since 1959. Complete responses range up to 75% and have induced curative responses in 11% of patients [14,21]. Regimens and formulation preferences vary by center; however, once-nightly application to the entire body from the neck down, sparing the intertriginous areas, is the generally accepted practice. In some cases, twice-daily applications may be indicated. Patients are encouraged to apply the NM at night to prevent contamination of the household environment and to limit contact with infants, small children, and pregnant women while the medication is on the skin. It may be removed in the bath or shower the following morning, followed by an emollient or topical steroid regimen. Patients applying the medication do not need to wear gloves, but caregivers are encouraged to wear chemotherapy gloves or a similar substitute that provides protection from absorption of the chemotherapy agent. Care should be taken to avoid getting the NM around or in the eye, and thorough hand washing is encouraged after application to prevent accidental contamination or ingestion. Systemic effects are minimal, because there is very little to no significant systemic absorption [22]. Empty medication containers should be disposed of in proper chemotherapeutic waste receptacles. The main side effects are irritant or allergic dermatitis (incidence is reduced with the gel and ointment bases) and carcinogenic potential, especially for squamous cell skin cancer, primarily in heavily pretreated skin (ie, skin exposed to prior radiation or PUVA treatments) [10,22]. Vigilant skin cancer checks are especially important for patients using this therapy.

Despite the efficacy of NM in early-stage disease and its relatively few side effects, several disadvantages exist. In recent years, the cost of NM has increased greatly, making it a very expensive therapy when applied daily to the entire body. Additionally, it must be compounded in the gel or petrolatum formulations by specialty pharmacists. In many cases, patients must first pay out of pocket for the medication and then try to seek reimbursement from their insurance plans. Some patients describe an alienation from their spouses because direct contact must be avoided at bedtime hours. It is important to broach lifestyle/quality-of-life issues with patients and provide suggestions on how to maintain desired spousal/significant other relationships with the least amount of interference from therapeutic requirements.

Topical retinoids

Bexarotene gel is the first topical retinoid approved by the FDA for use in CTCL. Although the exact mechanism of action is unknown, it is thought that both oral and topical retinoids act to induce apoptosis, decrease cell proliferation, increase cell differentiation, and modulate T-cell immunity [14]. In 67 patients who had stage IA–IIA CTCL, a phase I–II clinical trial demonstrated a 21% complete response rate and a 42% partial response rate [23]. Bexarotene gel is applied only to affected lesions, generally in limited areas, because it is routinely irritating to the skin. Before application, the normal skin surrounding the treated lesion should be protected with a coat of petroleum jelly. To a certain extent, this lesional irritation is a desired effect. The irritation, however, can be come very severe, requiring a holiday from its use and topical steroid applications to sooth the irritant effect. Application regimens must be individualized according to patient tolerance of the drug. Alternating regimens, such as every other day or 2 days on/1 day off, may help the patient tolerate the irritation and gradually build up to longer intervals of use. Again, expense is an issue in prescribing this drug.

Radiation therapy

Radiation therapy is another mainstay of therapy for CTCL, because the neoplastic T cells are among the most sensitive to radiation. Radiation therapy is documented as one of the earliest therapeutic options used, beginning in 1902 [24,25]. Extensive plaque and tumor lesions are treated most commonly with radiation, using either local delivery of radiation to specific target lesions (spot treatment) or, for more extensive plaque- or tumor-stage disease, total body skin electron beam (TBSEB) therapy. TBSEB requires specialized radiation oncology centers capable of delivering radiation to entire body fields. A typical treatment regimen provides a total dose of 3000 to 3600 Gy administered over a 9- to 10-week period with a 1-week rest period in the middle of the regimen [25]. This regimen may be adapted further because of multiple circumstances, including the patient's tolerance to the regimen and ability to travel almost daily to the specialty center. Some patients who do not live within driving distance choose to move near the treatment center temporarily and take advantage of hospital-associated reduced-rate housing. This option, although very demanding and expensive for the patient and family, helps increase compliance, decrease fatigue, and reduce associated stress. This is one therapy in which practitioners warn patients, "You probably will get worse before you get better," because there are several common side effects from the TBSEB. These side effects include nail and hair loss, eye irritation/dryness, inability to sweat, skin irritation [25] that at times is severe enough to produce significant pain, immobility, extremity edema, and interference with activities of daily living. When side effects of this severity occur, a break from therapy helps patients recover and then resume treatments. Spot treatments are tolerated more easily, although some degree of skin irritation still can occur.

Antibiotic therapy

The prophylactic use of topical antibacterial agents may be helpful in decreasing bacterial or fungal colonization on the skin. Bathing in a Dakin's solution (sodium hypochlorite) or a vinegar solution will help decrease bacteria. For fungal overgrowth, a capful of gentian violet in the bath or Castelani's paint topically only to affected areas may be helpful. Caution is necessary during application, because gentian violet and Castelani's paint will stain skin, clothing, bathroom fixtures, and other exposed items.

Systemic therapy

Extracorporeal photochemotherapy

Extracorporeal photochemotherapy (ECP) or photopheresis is a novel therapy approved by the FDA in 1987 for the palliative treatment of the skin manifestations of CTCL [26]. In the landmark study that established FDA approval of ECP, 27 of 37 patients who had refractory disease (73%) responded with improved skin scores [27]. A long-term follow-up study of this same group of patients demonstrated a doubled median survival of 60.3 months, as compared with previous median survival data of 30 months in patients who had similar clinical features [28]. ECP involves a pheresis procedure in which a fraction of the patient's white blood cells are separated by centrifugation, collected in a photoactivation chamber over a three- to six-cycle collection phase, then photoactivated with UVA light using the photosensitizing agent methoxsalen injected directly into the collected white blood cells. The treated cells are exposed to a predetermined dose of UVA light outside the body (extracorporeally) and then are returned to the patient through an established venous access (Fig. 9). ECP most commonly is done as an outpatient procedure on 2 consecutive days one time per month. Accelerated therapy, given every 2 weeks, may be indicated for patients who have SzS and exfoliative erythroderma. Because this therapy must be provided in a hospital or outpatient clinic setting,

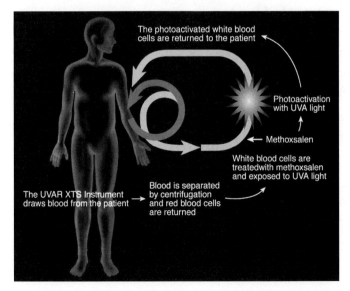

Fig. 9. Extracorporeal photopheresis process. (THERAKOS Photopheresis. Reprinted with permission of THERAKOS, Inc.)

insurance plans should cover the high cost of therapy. It is not offered routinely in all major hospital settings, requiring some patients to travel far distances to receive treatment (Fig. 10).

The mechanism of action remains unclear after nearly 20 years since its approval and widespread use. The treatment of the white blood cells with activated methoxsalen results in apoptosis of the treated cells. Once reinfused back into the patient, these apoptotic cells are processed within the patient's body, inducing a chain of immunologic events. Foss [29] summarizes it in this way: "The evolving model for the mechanism of action of ECP is that it is the ingestion of apoptotic T-cells, which initiates the process of activation and cytokine secretion by antigen-presenting cells, which subsequently leads to generation of tolerogenic dendritic cells and subsequently a regulatory T-cell response."

ECP is best initiated through peripheral venous access using a 16- or 17-gauge dialysis-type catheter to promote adequate blood flow during each collection cycle, which requires about 1 pint of blood for processing of the white blood cells. The entire procedure takes about 3 hours, on average, to complete. Patients must protect themselves from UVL exposure for 24 hours after each treatment, as described previously for PUVA.

Side effects related to ECP are mild and transient. Bruising, bleeding, hematoma, local infection, and thrombophlebitis are risks associated with any

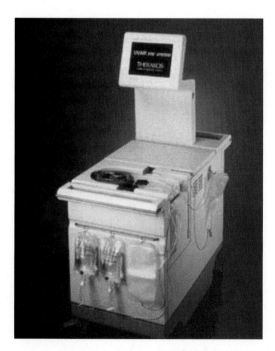

Fig. 10. Extracorporeal photopheresis instrument. (THERAKOS UVAR XTS Photopheresis System. Reprinted with permission of THERAKOS, Inc.)

intravenous procedure. If peripheral venous access is inadequate, a central catheter or high-flow implanted port may be required. These techniques must be used cautiously, and the risk/benefit ratio of treatment must be considered carefully, because the risks of serious infections and septicemia are increased in patients who have erythroderma and SzS [10]. Hypotension and hypovolemia may develop in some individuals who have low body weight or anemia. These conditions are reversed with the infusion of additional fluids and Trendelenburg positioning. Low-grade fever and transient increase in erythema and itching may develop 6 to 8 hours after the procedure. This manifestation may indicate an immunologic response following reinfusion of the treated cells. Patients who are susceptible to fluid volume shifts (eg, patients who have congestive heart failure) may experience exacerbation of the congestive heart failure symptoms if they are unable to handle approximately 500 to 600 mL of additional fluids delivered during the ECP procedure. These patients may require additional diuretics to offset the positive fluid balance.

Denileukin diftitox

Denileukin diftitox is a fusion protein approved by the FDA in 1998 for recurrent CTCL. The drug consists of two fused parts: an interleukin-2 cytokine and the diphtheria toxin. Specifically targeted for T cells expressing the CD25 antibody, the interleukin-2 portion of the protein attaches to the activated T cell; once the drug is inside the cell, the inactivated diphtheria toxin is released to inhibit protein synthesis and, ultimately, cause cell death [10].

Denileukin diftitox must be administered in a hospital-based clinic or outpatient chemotherapy center where emergency support services are available. It is given, at least initially, for 5 days every 3 weeks. Standard doses are 9 or 18 µg/kg, and premedication with oral corticosteroids, diphenhydramine, and acetaminophen is recommended . The three most common side effects are (1) flulike symptoms (fever/chills, muscle/joint aches, nausea, diarrhea, headache, asthenia), which are most prevalent during the first two cycles of therapy and diminish over time; (2) hypersensitivity reactions (hypotension, dyspnea, chest pain, back pain, vasodilation, rash); and (3) vascular leak syndrome (VLS) with resultant hypoalbuminemia, hypotension, and edema. VLS may occur in up to 25% of patients [30]. In the author's experience, VLS seems to be more prevalent in older patients or those who have a high tumor burden. It may be severe enough to warrant hospitalization and/or admission to the ICU for careful fluid and pulmonary management. Patients should be weighed daily during therapy and at home during the off-treatment interval. A weight gain of more than 1.5 kg during the week of drug infusion is cause to hold therapy and observe carefully for signs of developing VLS. Additionally, patients should be instructed to eat a diet high in protein to help maintain intravascular albumin levels. In accordance with the product insert, patients should report any visual changes, because in postmarketing data collection some patients reported visual disturbances [31].

Once again, the cost of denileukin diftitox is extremely high. Most insurance programs do cover the drug because it must be delivered in a clinic/hospital setting, and a patient-assistance program is available through the manufacturer to assist patients with noncovered expenses (see the section in this article titled "Support and Patient Resources").

Retinoids and vitamin A derivatives

Retinoids and vitamin A derivatives include isotretinoin (more commonly used) and acitretin. Although the exact mechanism of action is unclear, it is known that they regulate cell differentiation and proliferation without causing immunosuppression [32]. Retinoids commonly are combined with other therapies, such as PUVA, interferon, and photopheresis, to treat CTCL. Extreme caution must be used to avoid pregnancy during retinoid use because they are known teratogens [10]. The most common adverse effects are dry skin and mucous membranes and hyperlipidemia. These effects can be ameliorated with extensive lubrication, antilipemics such as gemfibrozil, and/or dose reductions.

Bexarotene is a synthetic retinoid X receptor (RXR)–selective retinoid, a retinoid subclass called "rexinoid," approved for CTCL by the FDA in 1999. As with the gel formulation, its mechanism of action is thought to be antiproliferative and apoptotic and to work through selective binding and activation of RXR receptors [33]. Bexarotene is taken daily at an average oral dose of 300 mg/m^2, although doses may be titrated up gradually to improve tolerance and obtain a therapeutic response. Common side effects include hypertriglyceridemia and central hypothyroidism and must be monitored by monthly blood evaluations. Antilipemic agents and thyroid supplementation are commonly required, along with dietary changes to limit fat and excess carbohydrate intake. Multiagent antilipemics still may be required to control lipid levels. Gemfibrozil is contraindicated as an antilipemic agent because it increases blood concentrations of bexarotene [14]. Less common side effects include neutropenia, liver function abnormalities, and headaches. An additional limitation to the use of oral bexarotene is its cost.

Interferons

Interferons are biologic response modifiers. Their effects are antiproliferative, cytotoxic, and immunomodulating. Interferon-α is used most commonly as a monotherapy in early-stage disease or in combination therapy for all stages. Interferon has been combined with PUVA, retinoids, photopheresis, and chemotherapy regimens with varying response rates [14]. The drug almost always is given by subcutaneous injection. Patients can readily be taught to self-inject interferon; however, some patients who cannot get prescription coverage for the drug may be able to get medical coverage for it when the injection is administered within a hospital or physician-run clinic. Doses used in CTCL are relatively low, with the average being between 3 and 5 MU three times per week. The side effects at this range are more tolerable but still can be difficult. They include flulike symptoms of fever/chills, muscle/joint aches, malaise, and fatigue. The flulike symptoms tend to diminish as tolerance to the drug develops over time. Adequate hydration, taking the injection at bedtime, and premedication with acetaminophen may help lessen side effects [10]. Anorexia is also a common side effect, with resultant weight loss that persists throughout drug use. Hematologic effects include elevated liver function tests and thrombocytopenia and neutropenia that improve or resolve with dose reduction.

Histone deacetylase inhibitors

In October, 2006 the FDA approved vorinostat, an antineoplastic agent, for primary CTCL that is progressive, persistent, or recurrent after two or more systemic therapies. Histone deacetylase inhibitors can induce tumor cell growth arrest, differentiation, or apoptosis [34]. In the single-arm study of 74 patients, stage IIB and higher, with 400 mg/d dosing, an overall objective response rate of 29.7% was seen. Median time to response was about 2 months, and response duration is estimated to exceed 6 months. Common side effects seen in the study were nausea and vomiting, weight loss, anorexia, diarrhea, constipation, fatigue, chills, thrombocytopenia, anemia, dysgeusia (taste alterations), and dry mouth. The serious adverse events included pulmonary embolism (4.7%), squamous cell carcinoma (3.5%), and anemia (2.3%). Common laboratory abnormalities included elevated serum creatinine, glucose, and proteinuria [35].

The standard dose of vorinostat is 400 mg daily (with food) by mouth. Dose reduction to 300 mg/d may be indicated if side effects are intolerable. Hematology and chemistry laboratory results should be monitored every 2 weeks for 2 months at initiation of therapy and monthly thereafter. Hypomagnesia and hypokalemia should be corrected before dosing. Despite its safe cardiac profile, baseline and periodic ECGs should be obtained to monitor the QTc interval. Patients should be instructed to report excessive vomiting or diarrhea, stay well hydrated by drinking quality liquids in the amount of eight 8-oz glasses/day, and report signs and symptoms of deep vein thrombosis and abnormal bleeding. Patients also should be cautioned about not opening or crushing the capsules [35]. Vorinostat also is an expensive drug, but currently there is a patient-assistance program entitled "ACT," to assist patients as needed.

Alemtuzumab

Alemtuzumab is a human immunoglobulin G1 anti-CD52 monoclonal antibody with an immunologic mechanism of action and is approved by the FDA only for B-cell chronic lymphocytic leukemia. It recently is receiving more attention for treatment of patients who have CTCL, especially those who have SzS and advanced-stage disease recalcitrant to most other available therapies. It has pan–immune system effects and binds to nearly all B- and T-cell lymphomas. Problematically, it produces extensive immuno-suppression, resulting in opportunistic infections and sepsis in some patients. Cardiac toxicity also has been noted [14]. It may be given intravenously or subcutaneously on an outpatient basis in varying regimens aimed at maximizing response and limiting immunologic devastation. Because of the potential for profound immunosuppression, patients should receive prophylactic antibacterial and antifungal coverage and observe basic neutropenic precautions as laboratory monitoring indicates.

Antibiotic therapy

Antibiotic therapy may be helpful in patients who have superinfections of bacterial toxins, especially staphylococcal enterotoxin. Recent discoveries demonstrated that staphylococcal enterotoxin stimulates the growth of malignant T cells through a novel mechanism of cross talk between malignant and nonmalignant T cells [36]. This finding is significant, because patients who have CTCL, especially those afflicted with erythrodermic MF or SzS, may be infected with staphylococcus in the skin and/or blood. Exacerbation of symptoms may be attributed to disease progression; however, it may be related more closely to patients' inability to clear the staphylococcal enterotoxin from the skin. Rapid improvement can be seen in some patients after antibiotic therapy. Therefore, it is important to consider the infectious component of CTCL when planning therapy [37].

Other therapies

The CTCL treatment armamentarium includes a long list of other therapies, including chemotherapy, bone marrow transplantation, and experimental therapies. Chemotherapy should be reserved for advanced relapsed or refractory disease when other immunologic and standard therapies have failed or for patients who have advanced nodal or visceral involvement at presentation [38]. Some of these other therapies are briefly summarized in Table 1 [39].

Nursing notes

Treatment goals should be established with the patient and discussed openly to determine the best treatment plan. If the patient is unwilling to undergo potentially remittive treatment and prefers a more palliative approach, therapy choices may be different. The patient's willingness and ability to comply with the treatment plan should be discussed. Potential limiting factors, such as cultural beliefs, lack of transportation, funds, insurance coverage, or physical ability to perform the required treatments will influence the choice of therapy.

Throughout the illness, patients often encounter an extensive list of choices of single or combination treatment options that frequently are exhausting and time-consuming and nearly always are expensive. These treatment issues have a consistent and cumulative impact on the patient's quality of life and go hand-in-hand with a patient's ability to maintain compliance with the treatment plan. With open and ongoing dialogue, the patient becomes a partner in the care plan rather than an object of it and is much more likely to be honest about his/her feelings regarding the treatment plan. The result can be increased compliance and improved outcomes.

Nursing role

Nursing care is a critical element to the successful care of patients who have CTCL and involves administering hands-on care, acting as the patient's advocate, and educating the patient and family members on a multitude of topics. The nurse is instrumental as a liaison with the physician, other health care providers (oncologist, radiation oncologist, dietician, and pharmacist), social services, community agencies, and family members. The author has found that patients are comfortable approaching the nurse with questions and concerns and consult the nurse as the first step in the process of seeking help. This awesome responsibility never ceases to amaze, and with it comes accountability to the patient who is entrusting the nurse to act on the information or question in the most appropriate manner. This type of relationship develops over time, but it is one of the most rewarding a nurse can experience.

One of the nurse's most important roles is to act as an advocate for the patient. As a patient advocate, it is necessary to attempt to see the disease through the patient's eyes. In this way, the nurse can understand what questions patients are not asking and then ask those questions for them, realize what help they do not have, but need, and then work to obtain that help for them, feel the symptom they are suffering and investigate its relief, and consider what they might be afraid to discuss and gently bring those issues to the forefront. Table 2 provides a summary of nursing care.

Because of the chronic nature of CTCL, troublesome symptoms, disruptive treatment regimens, and alteration in body image, many affected patients report significant impact on their quality of life. A recent study supported by the Cutaneous Lymphoma Foundation (CLF) used a four-page self-administered questionnaire sent to 930 patient-members of the CLF. The response rate was 68%, and 89% of the respondents reported having MF. This survey revealed multiple areas affecting health-related quality of life among respondents. Table 3 provides a selected summary [8]. These survey results have important implications for nurses and physicians in assuring that patient's concerns regarding quality of life are addressed as part of the plan of care.

Table 1
Summary of additional treatments for cutaneous T-cell lymphoma

Treatment name	Regimen	Patient education/Nursing care
Bone marrow transplantation	Limited experience Best results with matched allogeneic transplants	Reserved for advanced, recalcitrant disease in younger patients able to tolerate myeloablative regimens
Methotrexate	Low-dose oral administration best tolerated More effective in stage III and IV and in combination with other agents	Monthly monitoring of hematology and chemistry is required Avoid alcohol, aspirin, nonsteroidal anti-inflammatory agents
Cyclophosphamide	Alkylating agent Daily oral dosing	Bladder toxicity and anemia are common side effects Monthly monitoring of hematology and chemistry is required Adequate daily hydration is necessary to prevent bladder complications
Gemcitabine	Given intravenously weekly for 2 or 3 weeks of a 4 week cycle	Common side effects include nausea or vomiting, fatigue, and flulike syndrome (fever, chills, muscle aches, headache) Bone marrow suppression and hair thinning can occur Rarely, constipation, diarrhea, or mouth sores
Pegylated doxorubicin	Given intravenously every 2 to 4 weeks	Immediate reactions include itching, hives, or a red rash at the injection site and along the vein, acute hypersensitivity reactions Mild nausea, pink/red urine for up to 48 hours after treatment Other effects include bone marrow suppression, increased sensitivity, redness, and desquamation of palms/soles Cardiac toxicity is dose related and must be followed with multigated angiograms or echocardiograms to monitor heart function

Pentostatin	Given intravenously every 1 to 2 weeks as single or combination therapy in advanced stages	Early side effects include nausea, vomiting, decreased appetite, diarrhea, headache, fatigue and cough Bone marrow suppression, increased infections, transient abnormal liver function, eyes and/or ear complaints, or rash and sensitivity to light may occur
Depsipeptide	HDAC inhibitor Intravenous infusion weekly for 3 weeks of 4-week cycle	Phase II clinical trial
Zanolimumab	Anti-CD4 antibody Intravenous infusion weekly for 12 weeks	Phase II clinical trial
Dendritic cell vaccine	Intra–lymph node vaccine derived from autologous mature dendritic cells loaded with tumor antigens	Phase II clinical trial
CLBH589B2201	HDAC inhibitor Oral agent dosed M-W-F	Phase II clinical trial

Abbreviations: HDAC, histone deacetylase; M-W-F, Monday, Wednesday, and Friday.
Data from Refs. [14,38,39].

Table 2
Nursing care

Identified problem ⇨ Expected outcomes	Essential nursing interventions/Patient education
Altered skin integrity: scaling, ulcerated plaques, tumors, fissuring, excoriations ⇨ Moisturized, intact skin integrity with no evidence of infection	Assess skin routinely for
	Open wounds
	Fissuring
	Excoriations (evidence of scratching)
	Extent of scaling/dryness
	Extremity edema
	Drainage, crusting, oozing
	Implement skin care
	Assist with application of topical regimen
	Use nonadherent dressings for any open, ulcerated wounds and use caution in removing old dressings to avoid pain and tissue loss
	Use caution in removing tape or avoid its use whenever possible because skin tears easily; stockinette to hold dressing in place on extremities works well and avoids use of tape
	Consider topical antibacterial medications for open areas
	Elevate edematous extremities
	Position and turn any immobile patient to avoid further skin breakdown and consider specialty beds or mattress overlays for patients at high risk for skin breakdown
	Teach basic skin care
	Maintain skin hydration with oral fluids and emollients, which help restore skin barrier and act as a protective layer
	Use warm water (hydrates skin) not hot (dries out skin) in bath or shower (lasting 10–20 minutes)
	Pat dry then apply emollients/other topical agents as prescribed—best absorbed when skin is slightly moist

Inability to maintain homeostasis ⇔ Comfort established and body temperature maintained

Use mild nonsoap products for cleansing or mild, moisturizing soaps; avoid harsh products (antibacterial soaps) or irritating clothing (wool)

Report open wounds, fever/chills, skin oozing or crusting

To create an antibacterial bath, add one fourth cup of household bleach, 1 cup of vinegar, or Dakin's solution to the bath water; this will help decrease bacterial counts on the skin

Maintain comfort and homeostasis

Keep room warm, free of drafts; provide extra blankets

Monitor temperature and maintain vigilance in monitoring for infections because signs may be masked by hypothermic state

Instruct patient to

Report change in temperature, signs of infection, or other constitutional symptoms (even low-grade fever may indicate infection in hypothermic patient)

Avoid exposure to extreme temperatures

Layering of clothing can help maintain body temperature

Pruritus ⇔ Decrease in pruritus rating with improved quality of life

Assist with antipruritic measures

Administer antipruritics

Moisturize skin often with emollients/prescribed regimen

Interrupt scratch/itch cycle by applying cool soaks or ice packs or encourage lukewarm bath/shower followed by re-moisturization

Oatmeal baths or mentholated/cooling lotions to calm skin

Offer distraction such as talking, walking, activity

Teach patient about

Side effects of antihistamines, especially sedating effects of common agents (diphenhydramine, doxepin—best used at night) alternating with nonsedating agents (loratadine, cetirizine) during day

Using caution in driving/activity until effect is known; being alert for increased risk of falling, especially in elderly

Importance of breaking scratch/itch cycle: explore what might work for each individual and plan alternative actions when itching becomes unbearable

Humidifying home during winter months with commercial humidifier or simple container of water placed near heat register

(continued on next page)

Table 2 (*continued*)

Identified problem ⇨ Expected outcomes	Essential nursing interventions/Patient education
	Avoiding the use of back-scratching devices, door jams, or other improvised, sharp objects to scratch self
	Keeping fingernails short to avoid unnecessary trauma and avoiding excessive rubbing with washcloths during bath; rubbing will thicken skin further and cause trauma
Skin pain ⇨ Improved pain rating	Ensure adequate pain relief
	Assess pain using 10-point pain scale, administer pain medications as ordered, and assess effectiveness of pain relief
	Assess for infection because infection may increase/instigate pain
	Culture wounds if infection is suspected and treat as indicated
	Provide other pain relief measures: position change, pillows, cold/warm compresses, massage, topical applications, distraction
	Consider need for special dressings, beds, or bed cradle to keep pressure off of painful skin
	Review with patient
	Use of pain scale as a measurement of pain
	Importance of reporting pain so that it can be adequately addressed and treated
	Avoidance of irritants, sharp fingernails/objects that will traumatize skin further
	Use of nonrestrictive, nonirritating clothing to avoid further discomfort/trauma
Decreased dexterity/mobility related to fissuring or hyperkeratosis of palms/soles, deconditioning, extremity edema ⇨ Able to perform activities of daily living at maximum potential	Assist with activities of daily living
	Assess level of independence and risk for falls
	Obtain physical therapy consult for use of assistive devices such as a walker, cane, wheel chair as needed, especially if fall risk is identified
	Obtain occupational therapy consult for use of adaptive devices (ie, bottle/can openers, large-grip fork/spoon)
	Encourage active range of motion or provide passive range of motion if needed
	Assess need for home care and provide referral
	Discuss with patient
	Applying gloves or socks after topical regimens may help intensify effect and relief to hands and feet; gloves also act as a protection for hands and may provide additional dexterity
	Using caution in bath/shower because topical products may produce slippery conditions
	Taking precautions to avoid falls: keeping night light on at night, sitting on edge of bed for several minutes before standing, using good slippers for support/traction, avoiding use of throw rugs

Anger, anxiety, fear, depression related to diagnosis ⇨ Exhibits effective coping mechanisms, participates in work, social, family functions

Maintain open communications
  Discuss concerns openly and honestly and encourage expression of feelings; involve family members as appropriate
  Provide time for questions and discussion of feelings
  Assess need for psychologic, spiritual, or caregiver support and make referrals as necessary
  Explain all procedures and rationales for therapies
  Assess coping strategies and provide positive reinforcement for positive behaviors; set limits on negative behaviors
  Involve patient in decision making
  Provide access to caregivers and offer reassurance of available help you are offering
Reinforce with patient
  Availability of caregivers and how to contact medical staff at any time of day/night
  Resources available for support within community or through the internet
  Demonstrate relaxation techniques and provide reading list of self help literature
  Review information provided by physician to assure understanding (ie, progress reports, laboratory reports, medications, and treatments)

Nutritional and metabolic deficiencies ⇨ Nutrition adequate to meet metabolic needs

Monitor fluid and electrolyte balance and ensure adequate nutrition
  Assess intake and output, weight gain/loss, edema
  Evaluate laboratory values for albumin, protein, iron, hemoglobin, hematocrit, red blood cell deficiencies
  Consult dietician as indicated
  Monitor dietary intake to determine actual needs and provide dietary supplements
Instruct patient about
  Need for nutritional supplements with loss of skin and accelerated metabolism of erythrodermic states
  Importance of high-protein, high-quality carbohydrate diet to maintain nutritional needs
  How meal planning may help to ensure adequate intake
  Reporting weight changes and extremity edema

(continued on next page)

Table 2 (*continued*)

Identified problem ⇨ Expected outcomes	Essential nursing interventions/Patient education
Socioeconomic limitations ⇨ Receives prescribed therapy	Advocate for patient's best interests
	Openly discuss issues related to abilities to comply with prescribed regimen (fiscally and physically)
	Write letters as needed for insurance approvals and assist with assistance applications (usually require brief information on diagnosis, prescribed therapy, physician signature)
	Act as liaison with primary care physicians, insurance representatives, social and community services to obtain needed referrals and services
	Provide referrals to support agencies as needed
	Assess need for home care services (nursing, home-health aide, palliative or hospice care)
	Empower patients and family members
	Provide information on national and local support services and available funds or other support through industry or nonprofit agencies
	Discuss use of hospital-based housing for prolonged therapy (TBSEB treatment protocols), patient assistance programs and agencies that offer support
	Explore acceptable alternative therapies or clinical trials that may fit into the patient's physical/financial abilities
Knowledge deficit related to disease process and treatment regimens ⇨ Demonstrates appropriate knowledge base to enhance compliance	Establish knowledge base with patient
	Assess readiness to learn about CTCL and provide depth of information as indicated by patient feedback and nonverbal cues
	Set aside time at each visit or encounter to discuss disease process and treatment regimens: purpose, side effects, dose, administration or application instructions, any safety measures (such as monitoring laboratory values), and when to call with problems
	Provide patient with multiple sources of written handouts from institution, industry, Web-based, agency pamphlets

Explain all procedures before implementing steps
Routinely assess understanding of information exchange
Ask patient and/or family to repeat back information and discuss how the treatment goals will be incorporated at home.
Demonstrate procedures and ask for return demonstrations
Provide time to assimilate information
Discuss realistic treatment expectations as another way to determine understanding and synthesis of information
Encourage positive self image
Discuss patient's perception of self and self-esteem
Take time to know the person beneath the skin and provide positive reinforcement for inner beauty, talents, life experiences and accomplishments
Encourage positive self-image and provide emotional support for distressing body image changes
Refer for additional emotional support as needed with psychiatry or counseling services
Explore ways to enhance self image
Encourage use of cosmetic camouflage with makeup, hairstyles, or clothing choices
Refer to specialty hair salon for styling or wig/hair salon for alopecia issues

Alteration in self-image ⇨ Demonstrates positive self-image and coping mechanisms

Abbreviation: TBSEB, total body skin electron beam.

Table 3
Selected summary of survey results on quality of life for patients who have cutaneous T-cell lymphoma

Importance of quality-of-life aspect	% Respondents indicating importance
Bothered by skin redness	94
Bothered by itching	88
Bothered by some pain	41
Bothered by "quite a bit" to "very much" pain	13
Bothered by skin scaling	83
Extent of symptoms affecting choice of clothes	63
Tired because of disease	66
Sleep affected	66
Feel ashamed because of disease	39
Feel unattractive	62
Affected sex life	47
Worry about seriousness of disease	94
Worry about dying	80
Feel financially burdened	61

Data from Demierre M, Gan S, Jones J, Miller D. Significant impact of cutaneous T-cell lymphoma on patient's quality of life: results of a 2005 National Cutaneous Lymphoma Foundation survey. Cancer 2006;107(10):2504–11.

Support and patient resources

The CLF was established in 1998 and formerly was known as the "Mycosis Fungoides Foundation." The CLF is dedicated to supporting people diagnosed as having a cutaneous lymphoma by promoting awareness and education, advancing patient care, and facilitating research. Among its many programs, the CLF partners with industry sponsors and medical centers to promote educational forums around the country through Web casts and day-long symposiums. It also provides two on-line support groups, one geared primarily for patients and one for parents of children diagnosed as having a cutaneous lymphoma. The CLF Website, www.clfoundation.org, is a rich resource of information on disease aspects, treatment options, diagnostic and treatment centers, and educational and advocacy projects.

Other online sources of information and support include

- American Academy of Dermatology (www.aad.org)
- American Cancer Society (www.cancer.org)
- CancerCare (www.cancercare.org)
- Dermatology Nurses Association (www.dnanurse.org)
- Lymphoma Research Foundation (www.lymphoma.org)
- National Cancer Institute (www.cancer.gov)
- National Coalition for Cancer Survivorship (www.canceradvocacy.org)
- The Leukemia and Lymphoma Society (www.lls.org)
- Patient Access Network Foundation (www.patientaccessnetwork.org)

The Patient Access Network Foundation is nonprofit organization dedicated to assisting insured patients who cannot afford the out-of-pocket costs of their required therapy. There is a specific fund for qualified patients who have CTCL. A financial application and physician documentation of disease are required to begin the process.

Nursing notes

The University of Pittsburgh Medical Center developed an annual educational and support meeting for patients and their family members. This group recently held the "Ninth Annual Brian V. Jegasothy Support Group for CTCL" in the fall of 2006 in partnership with the CLF. This meeting has been a model for establishing other support meetings held around the United States. There is an emphasis on creating a forum for exchanging and sharing basic and advanced information on cutaneous lymphomas among physician experts and patients. The meeting also allows patients and their caregivers to ask the expert questions in an informal setting, network with other patients, share practical pearls of wisdom, and offer one another general support.

Summary

CTCL is an uncommon and complex malignancy of the immune system with a wide range of clinical presentations primarily involving the skin. Involvement of lymph nodes and distant organs is also possible. The disease is chronic by nature and as such affords the dermatologist and dermatology nurse an opportunity to provide care for the patient on a long-term basis. An extensive menu of skin-directed and/or systemic treatment options exists. Best practices in management involve multidisciplinary collaboration. Nursing care for patients who have CTCL is a critical component in the successful management of the disease and requires special attention to the patient's physical, emotional, and spiritual needs. Nurses can make a significant impact by being accessible, offering emotional support, demonstrating advocacy, and providing ongoing education for the patient and family.

References

[1] Slater D. The new World Health Organization-European Organization for research and treatment of cancer classification for cutaneous lymphomas: a practical marriage of two giants. Br J Dermatol 2005;153:874–80.
[2] Girardi M, Heald P, Wilson L. The pathogenesis of mycosis fungoides. N Engl J Med 2004; 350(19):1978–88.
[3] Kim E, Hess S, Richardson S, et al. Immunopathogenesis and therapy of cutaneous T cell lymphoma. J Clin Invest 2005;115(4):798–812.

[4] Criscione VD, Weinstock MA. Incidence of cutaneous T-cell lymphoma in the United States, 1973–2002. Arch Dermatol 2007;143(7):854–9.

[5] Suarez-Varela Morales, Llopis-Gonzalez A, Marquina Vila A, et al. Mycosis fungoides: review of epidemiological observations. Dermatology 2000;201:21–8.

[6] Hodak E, Klein T, Gabay B, et al. Familial mycosis fungoides: report of 6 kindreds and a study of the HLA system. J Am Acad Dermatol 2005;53(3 pt 1):393–402.

[7] Zackheim HS, Amin S, Kashani-Saber M, et al. Prognosis in cutaneous T-cell lymphoma by skin stage: long term survival in 489 patients. J Am Acad Dermatol 1999;85:208–12.

[8] Demierre M, Gan S, Jones J, et al. Significant impact of cutaneous T-cell lymphoma on patient's quality of life: results of a 2005 national cutaneous lymphoma foundation survey. Cancer 2006;107(10):2504–11.

[9] Sterry W, Muche JM. Other systemic lymphomas with skin infiltration. In: Freedberg I, Eisen A, Wolff K, Austen KF, et al, editors. Fitzpatrick's dermatology in general medicine, vol. 2. 6th edition. New York: McGraw-Hill; 2003. p. 1558–67.

[10] Parker S, Bradley B. Treatment of cutaneous T-cell lymphoma/mycosis fungoides. Dermatol Nurs 2006;18(6):566–75.

[11] Vonderheid E, Bernengo M, Burg G, et al. Update on erythrodermic cutaneous T-cell lymphoma: report to the International Society for Cutaneous Lymphomas. J Am Acad Dermatol 2002;46:95–106.

[12] Kim Y, Liu H, Mraz-Gernhard S, et al. Long-term outcome of 525 patients with mycosis fungoides and Sezary syndrome: clinical prognostic factors and risk for disease progression. Arch Dermatol 2003;139(7):857–66.

[13] Kim YH, Hoppe RT. Mycosis fungoides and the Sezary syndrome. Semin Oncol 1999;26: 276–89.

[14] Apisarnthanarax N, Talpur R, Duvic M. Treatment of cutaneous T-cell lymphoma: current status and future directions. Am J Clin Dermatol 2002;3(3):193–215.

[15] Kim E, Lin J, Junkin-Hopkins J, et al. Mycosis fungoides and Sezary syndrome: an update. Curr Oncol Rep 2006;8:376–86.

[16] Vonderheid E. Treatment planning in cutaneous T-cell lymphoma. Dermatol Ther 2003;16: 276–82.

[17] Zackheim HS, Kashani-Sabet M, Amin S. Topical corticosteroids for mycosis fungoides: experience in 79 patients. Arch Dermatol 1988;134:949–54.

[18] Zackheim HS. Treatment of patch-stage mycosis fungoides with topical corticosteroids. Dermatol Ther 2003;16:283–7.

[19] Baron E, Stevens S. Phototherapy for cutaneous T-cell lymphoma. Dermatol Ther 2003;16: 303–10.

[20] Clark C, Dawe R, Evans A, et al. Narrowband TL-01 phototherapy for patch-stage mycosis fungoides. Arch Dermatol 2000;136:748–52.

[21] Vonderheid E, Tan E, Kantor A, et al. Long-term efficacy, curative potential and carcinogenicity of topical mechlorethamine chemotherapy in cutaneous T-cell lymphoma. J Am Acad Dermatol 1989;20:416–28.

[22] Kim Y. Management with topical nitrogen mustard in mycosis fungoides. Dermatol Ther 2003;16:288–98.

[23] Brenemen D, Duvic M, Kuzel T, et al. Phase I-II trial bexarotene gel for the skin-directed treatment of patients with cutaneous T-cell lymphoma. Arch Dermatol 2002;138: 325–32.

[24] Jones G, Hoppe R, Glatstein E. Electron beam treatment for cutaneous T-cell lymphoma. Hematol Oncol Clin North Am 1995;9:1057–75.

[25] Hoppe RT. Mycosis fungoides: radiation therapy. Dermatol Ther 2003;16:347–54.

[26] Weber R. Therapeutic/treatment modalities. In: Hill M, editor. Dermatologic nursing essentials: a core curriculum. 2nd edition. Pitman (NJ): Anthony J. Jannetti, Inc.; 2003. p. 74–9.

[27] Edelson R, Berger C, Gasparro F, et al. Treatment of cutaneous T-cell lymphoma by extracorporeal photochemotherapy. N Engl J Med 1987;316(6):297–303.

[28] Zic J, Stricklin G, Greer J, et al. Long term follow-up of patients with cutaneous T-cell lymphoma treated with extracorporeal photochemotherapy. J Am Acad Dermatol 1996; 35(6):935–45.

[29] Foss F. New insights into the mechanism of action of extracorporeal phototherapy. Transfusion 2006;46(1):6–8.

[30] Olsen E, Duvic M, Frankel A, et al. Pivotal phase III trial of two dose levels of denileukin diftitox for the treatment of cutaneous T-cell lymphoma. J Clin Oncol 2001;19(2):376–88.

[31] Denileukin Diftitox Product Insert (April 2007). Available at: www.eisai.com. Accessed April 15, 2007.

[32] Nguyen E-QH, Wolverton S. Systemic retinoids. In: Wolverton S, editor. Comprehensive dermatologic drug therapy. Philadelphia: W.B. Saunders; 2001. p. 269–310.

[33] Duvic M, Hymes K, Heald P, et al. Bexarotene is effective and safe for treatment of refractory advanced-stage cutaneous T-cell lymphoma: multinational phase II-III trial results. J Clin Oncol 2001;19(9):2456–71.

[34] Johnstone RW. Histone-deacetylase inhibitors: novel drugs for the treatment of cancer. Nat Rev Drug Discov 2003;1:287–99.

[35] PI slide kit. Available at: www.zolinza.com. Accessed December 10, 2006.

[36] Woetmann A, Lovato P, Eriksen K, et-al. Non-malignant T cells stimulate growth of T-cell lymphoma cells in the presence of bacterial toxins. Blood First Edition Paper, prepublished online 2006 DOI: 10.1182/Blood-2006-04-017863.

[37] Jackow CM, Cather JC, Hearne V, et al. Association of erythrodermic cutaneous T-cell lymphoma, superantigen-positive Staphylococcus aureus, and oligoclonal T-cell receptor V-beta gene expansion. Blood 1997;89:32–40.

[38] Kuzel T. Systemic chemotherapy for the treatment of mycosis fungoides and Sezary syndrome. Dermatol Ther 2003;16:355–61.

[39] Available at: www.clfoundation.org. Accessed December 10, 2006.

NURSING CLINICS
OF NORTH AMERICA

Nurs Clin N Am 42 (2007) 457–465

Using Angiogenesis in Chronic Wound Care with Becaplermin and Oxidized Regenerated Cellulose/Collagen

Clair Hollister, LVN[a],*, Vincent W. Li, MD[b,c]

[a]*Department of Dermatology, University of California, San Diego, 9350 Campus Point Drive, Suite 2B, La Jolla, CA 92037, USA*
[b]*Institute for Advanced Studies, The Angiogenesis Foundation, P.O. Box 382111, Cambridge, MA 02238, USA*
[c]*The Angiogenesis Clinic, Department of Dermatology, Brigham and Women's Hospital, 211 Longwood Avenue, Boston, MA 02115, USA*

For most of the last century, chronic wound care was a practice of passive techniques, designed to prevent the progression of the wound. The last decade, however, has seen a change in active wound care. These advanced techniques focus on improving the wound at the molecular level to accelerate wound healing. Successful modalities include tissue-engineered products, hyperbaric oxygen, negative pressure therapy, electrical stimulation, and recombinant growth factors [1–7]. This shift in the treatment of wound care saw the development of a recombinant human platelet-derived growth factor (rh PDGF-BB), approved by the Food and Drug Administration (FDA) for nonhealing diabetic ulcers in 1997 [8,9]. Now commonly used for treatment, becaplermin (REGRANEX) stimulates granulation and increases the incidence of complete wound closure [2,8–10]. Another development was found to protect growth factors and granulation tissue by inhibiting wound proteases [11]. This product is oxidized regenerated cellulose (ORC)/collagen (PROMOGRAN). Used together, an optimal environment for wound healing can be created.

Angiogenesis

Angiogenesis is simply the growth of new capillary blood vessels. The medical community is using what they know of angiogenesis to produce

---

* Corresponding author.
E-mail address: chollister@ucsd.edu (C. Hollister).

medications that stimulate or inhibit these molecular roles. Antiangiogenesis is the motivation behind many cancer-fighting treatments, just as angiogenesis is the factor behind many healing therapies. The focus of this article is how becaplermin and ORC/collagen are used to stimulate angiogenesis in chronic wound care.

Phases of wound healing

To emphasize the role of angiogenesis in wound healing, one must first look at the naturally occurring process of wound repair in a healthy individual. The three phases of wound healing are codependent and overlapping.

Phase I (inflammatory phase) occurs at time of injury and continues for approximately 5 days. Injury immediately kicks off the events that lead to clotting. A temporary increase in permeability of the vascular wall allows neutrophils, platelets, and plasma proteins to enter the wound. With the initial injury, cell membranes release vasoconstrictors that limit hemorrhaging. Platelets then release multiple chemokines that help stabilize the wound with clot formation. The second part of this phase starts when the platelets release growth factors that draw polymorphic neutrophils (PMNs) into the wound, initiating early inflammation. For about 48 hours, the PMNs keep the wound clean and prevent infection by killing bacteria and removing foreign debris. After 48 hours, the PMNs recruit macrophages into the wound to replace them slowly as the primary inflammatory cell. Both cells, the PMN's and macrophages, are releasing growth factors as they continue to maintain a clean wound [12,13].

Phase II (proliferation phase) occurs from day 4 to approximately day 21. This phase overlaps the first phase. It is characterized by epithelialization, angiogenesis, granulation tissue formation, and collagen deposition. Fibroblasts, recruited by growth factors, lay down new collagen that works with new blood vessel growth (codependent), allowing epithelial cells to traverse the wound, forming granulation tissue [12,13].

Phase III (maturation phase) overlaps phase II and can last for more than a year. It is characterized by wound contraction, resulting in a smaller amount of apparent scar tissue, as compared with the original wound size. The collagen is continually reorganizing during this time to get maximal tensile strength [12,13].

Growth factors

Growth factors are a large family of proteins designed to promote cell proliferation and migration. About 20 growth factors have been identified that stimulate angiogenesis [2]. Among these are platelet-derived growth factor (PDGF), vascular endothelial growth factor (VEGF), fibroblast growth factor (FGF), and the transforming growth factors [1].

One of the first cells in the wound is the platelet. Platelets are responsible for releasing many growth factors into the wound, including PDGF, which is unique because of its multiple roles in stimulating endothelial cells and stabilizing the new vasculature [14]. PDGF is released by platelets, macrophages, and monocytes, where it then binds to its receptor on the surface of endothelial cells. Binding activates signals that begin cell proliferation, migration, invasion, tube formation, and vascular survival [15–17].

PDGF promotes the release of the other growth factors including VEGF and FGF [2,18,19]. Studies have shown that when PDGF is combined with either VEGF or FGF, more functional blood vessels result [3,20].

Another way that PDGF impacts vascular stabilization is through its ability to recruit smooth muscle cells and pericytes to newly forming blood vessels [21–24]. This concept is important because diabetic ulcers have shown a diminished expression of PDGF [2,25]. One of the primary reasons becaplermin is so helpful in stimulating healing in diabetic wounds is that, in a sense, it serves as a type of gene-based therapy. Gene-based therapies offer the theoretic advantage of sustained local expression of growth factors to target tissues [1,26]. Later in this article, the important role of becaplermin in diabetic wound healing due to PDGF concepts is discussed.

Proteases

In the early inflammatory phase of wound healing, a family of enzymes called proteases is introduced into the wound. They are expressed transiently at the tip of newly forming blood vessels to facilitate vascular growth [2,27]. In normally healing wounds, proteases assist in tissue remodeling and removal of necrotic tissue. Chronic wounds have an excess of protease activity. When this level becomes abnormally elevated, proteases may destroy growth factors, inhibit angiogenesis, and break down granulation tissue [27]. Because of this phenomenon, controlling protease activity has become a key factor in managing a chronic wound.

Becaplermin

Becaplermin is the first, and currently only, recombinant angiogenic growth factor to become FDA approved and is widely used by wound care specialists [1,8,9]. Because it is a peptide drug, it needs to be stored in the refrigerator to prevent heat degradation. This drug attaches to the PDGF receptors in the wound bed to start angiogenesis. It is a gel that is applied topically and is easy for patients to use at home.

Through four multicenter, randomized, parallel-group clinical trials that evaluated the effects of once-daily topical becaplermin gel in 922 patients who had nonhealing diabetic foot ulcers of at least 8 weeks' duration, clinical efficacy was established [28]. These patients were randomly assigned to a standardized regimen of good wound care alone, or good wound care plus becaplermin gel or a placebo gel of sodium carboxymethylcellulose. Treatment continued for 20 weeks or until the wound healed, with the primary endpoint of complete healing, defined as 100% epithelialization with no drainage. Becaplermin gel significantly increased the incidence of complete healing compared with the placebo gel (50% compared with 35%), based on an analysis of patients with a baseline ulcer area common to all trials, representing 95% of all patients [1,28].

Oxidized regenerated cellulose/collagen

ORC/collagen is a medical dressing composed of freeze-dried ORC and bovine collagen [29]. This dressing binds and neutralizes destructive proteases in chronic wound fluid. Once the proteases are neutralized, they undergo an alteration of their protein configuration, which makes them inactive. The dressing then binds directly to growth factors and is capable of releasing them back into the wound over time while keeping the proteases inactive [30], which helps to protect PDGF and other growth factors like FGF and VEGF from destruction related to overly high levels of these proteases in the wound.

An important study documenting the efficacy of ORC/collagen dressings was performed, in vitro, by incubating exogenous PDGF with plasmin, a protease present in chronic wound fluid, in the presence of ORC/collagen. The PDGF activity was retained and showed the protective effect of this dressing [2,30]. An additional study incubated exogenous PDGF in chronic wound fluid for 24 hours at 37°C with either ORC/collagen or a standard gauze dressing [30]. Only the ORC/collagen group demonstrated significant recoverable PDFG activity after incubation. These studies support a mechanism by which ORC/collagen promotes angiogenesis by protecting growth factors [2].

Use of the ORC/collagen dressing is quite simple. It is cut to the size of the wound bed and gently pressed to the base. This dressing is followed in application by a secondary dressing to help maintain the moist wound environment. Once the ORC/collagen is affixed as described, it begins to absorb drainage, and over a period of days it dissolves and is completely reabsorbed into the wound.

Recognizing its ease of use and potential indications in wound care, recent advancements in ORC/collagen have taken place. One such advancement includes the introduction of ORC/collagen impregnated with silver (Promogran prisma). Quickly becoming the popular dressing of choice for infected or potentially infected wounds, silver products provide antisepsis to the chronic wound.

Becaplermin and oxidized regenerated cellulose/collagen combined

Creating regimens of care for chronic wounds using becaplermin and ORC/collagen includes many options. In the authors' clinic, they combine the use of becaplermin with ORC/collagen to enhance growth factor efficacy. Combining them is designed to

- Deliver a potent growth factor to stimulate wound granulation
- Optimize the growth factor's effect by protecting it from degradation by proteases

The authors have developed a protocol implementing the optimal methods of treating the patient with becaplermin and ORC/collagen.

Wound evaluation

The evaluation of all chronic wounds includes assessment for presence of infection, determination of primary cause, assessment of nutritional status, and assessment of macrovascular and microvascular disease. Any suspicion that a cutaneous malignancy, vasculitis, or thromboembolic cause may be present requires a biopsy to be performed before initiating treatment. This step is very important because becaplermin accelerates angiogenesis in all cells, thus facilitating growth in malignant cells.

Initiation of treatment

If several weeks of routine conventional management of the acute wound have not resulted in improvement, or in the case of a chronic wound, the authors select an advanced modality to accelerate closure. Because granulation tissue is needed universally, they consider becaplermin for almost every patient. Their experience has shown that the earlier becaplermin treatment is initiated, the faster wound closure is achieved, regardless of wound cause.

Additionally, the use of ORC/collagen is generally optimal for almost every patient who has such wounds. The only patients not considered are those with known allergies to any related collagen products. Also, for patients who have a high potential for infection, the addition of ORC/collagen with silver provides an added antiseptic benefit.

Debridement

Prior to adding either becaplermin or ORC/collagen to the wound care regimen, the wound base must first be prepared. Appropriate, sharp debridement is essential to the successful use of becaplermin [31]. In the authors' clinic, sterile debridement is achieved by first cleansing the wound with an antiseptic surgical soap. Debridement is performed by the physician with a number 15 scalpel blade, an iris scissors, or a curette to remove necrotic tissue or fibrinous slough, before initiation of growth factor therapy. When debridement is performed properly, it will produce some minor local bleeding at the wound bed. This bleeding can stimulate angiogenesis in response to the new accumulation of platelets and also by exposing the cellular receptors so that PDGF can activate vascular endothelial cells. Additionally, it serves to remove senescent cells that do not respond to growth factors, allowing the wound margins to close by changing a chronic wound into an acute wound.

Although sharp debridement is optimal for use with becaplermin, other options can be considered. For patients who are unable to tolerate sharp debridement, or for those with a large amount of adherent eschar, enzymatic debridement is an option. It is necessary first to score the eschar with a 15 blade to allow the enzymatic cream or ointment to start degrading the necrotic tissue.

Becaplermin

Next, the use of becaplermin, the first advanced modality, is implemented. Only a small amount of becaplermin is necessary to treat the entire wound surface. A small amount of the gel should be applied to a cotton-tipped applicator and spread thinly onto the wound surface, allowing the rh PDHF-BB (becaplermin) to come into direct contact with the exposed receptors.

Oxidized Regenerated Cellulose/collagen

ORC/collagen is the next layer to be applied. The ORC/collagen is cut to the size of the wound bed before application, which allows it to fit into the base of the wound and come into contact with all the growth factors and proteases. The same technique is also used for the ORC/collagen with silver. It should be gently pressed to the base of the wound to allow the material to conform to the concavity of the wound bed. An additional method involves applying a second layer of the becaplermin atop the ORC/collagen, which promotes a sustained release effect as the ORC/collagen is resorbed into the wound. Finally, the focus turns to coordination of dressing changes.

Dressing changes

The original clinical trials for becaplermin involved twice-daily dressing changes, using saline to rinse the wound, as recommended by the package insert [2]. This high frequency of dressing changes is often impractical for patients and reduces patient compliance. In their clinic, the authors have seen positive results using less frequent dressing changes, once daily or every other day. Again, this frequency depends on the individual wound and the amount of drainage present. It is always necessary to maintain a moist wound environment on which hydrogels can be added below the ORC/collagen to maintain moisture. Some wounds have the potential of becoming too moist, leading to maceration of healthy tissue and an increase of bacterial bioburden, increasing the risk for infection. In these instances, it is recommended that the patient be treated instead with ORC/collagen with silver. If ORC/collagen with silver is used, it is necessary to rinse with sterile water to avoid neutralizing the silver ions. To help with excess moisture, one could also add an alginate or foam dressing after the ORC/collagen to absorb the excess drainage.

Added benefits

Using this treatment gives patients added benefits; not only does it accelerate healing and wound closure but is also cost effective. When a patient heals more quickly, he/she spends less money on dressing supplies and, for some patients, less on visiting nurses, which is always a major concern for patients and the health care industry as a whole. Another benefit is an increase in patient compliance. When patients are seeing improvement in their wound healing, they are more likely to continue with it. As all nurses are well aware, it is impossible to have successful healing without the patient being compliant with the wound care process.

Summary

Angiogenesis is part of the normal process of wound healing. Several factors help to regulate this healing process. Chronic wounds have defects in this normal process related to the underlying cause of the wound, whether diabetic, venous, or other. To bridge the defects in this process, science has been able to control part of the molecular process of angiogenesis, or new blood vessel growth, through the use of recombinant growth factors. Becaplermin has demonstrated its ability to provide that much-needed bridge to promote healing, dramatically improving patient wound outcomes. Becaplermin is currently the only FDA-approved growth factor for chronic wound healing, and as it bridges the gap of healing to promote angiogenesis it thus encourages an increase in granulation tissue.

Granulation tissue is required for wounds to heal, so becaplermin has a wide potential in the management of various wounds [2]. Becaplermin can be used alone or in combination with various other modalities, such as bioengineered tissue equivalents and negative pressure therapy. To enhance the applied growth factor effects, ORC/collagen can be applied with becaplermin to maximize the potential of both these products. With the recent advancement in biologically active dressings like ORC/collagen, one can control wound proteases and promote angiogenesis, thereby achieving the maximum benefit for patients and their healing wounds.

References

[1] Li WW, Li VW, Tsakayannis D. Angiogenesis in wound healing. Contemp Surg 2003;(Suppl):5–32.
[2] Li WW, Li VW. Therapeutic angiogenesis for wound healing. Wounds: A Compendium of Clinical Research and Practice 2003;15(Suppl 9):3–10.
[3] Richardson TP, Peters MC, Ennett AB, et al. Polymeric system for dual growth factor delivery. Nat Biotechnol 2001;19:1029–34.
[4] Jiang WG, Harding KG. Enhancement of wound tissue expansion and angiogenesis by matrix-embedded fibroblast (Dermagraft), a role of hepatocyte growth factor/scatter factor. Int J Mol Med 1998;2(2):203–10.

[5] Heng MC, Harker J, Csathy G, et al. Angiogenesis in necrotic ulcers treated with hyperbaric oxygen. Ostomy Wound Manage 2000;46(9):18–28, 30–2.

[6] Ingber DE, Prusty D, Sun Z, et al. Cell shape, cytoskeletal mechanics, and cell cycle control in angiogenesis. J Biomech 1995;28(12):1471–84.

[7] Chekanov V, Rayel R, Krum D, et al. Electrical stimulation promotes angiogenesis in a rabbit hind-limb ischemia model. Vasc Endovascular Surg 2002;36(5):357–66.

[8] Wieman TJ, Smiell JM, Su Y. Efficacy and safety of a topical gel formulation of recombinant human platelet-derived growth factor-BB (becaplermin) in patients with chronic neuropathic diabetic ulcers. A phase III randomized placebo-controlled double-blind study. Diabetes Care 1998;21:822–7.

[9] Li WW, Li VW, Tsakayannis D. Angiogenesis therapies. Concepts, clinical trials, and considerations for new drug development. In: Fan T-PD, Kohn EC, editors. The new angiotherapy. Totowa (NJ): Humana Press; 2001. p. 547–71.

[10] Bennett SP, Griffiths GD, Schor AM, et al. Growth factors in the treatment of diabetic foot ulcers. Br J Surg 2003;90(2):133–46.

[11] Veves A, Sheehan P, Pham HT. A randomized, controlled trial of promogran (a collagen/oxidized regenerated cellulose dressing) vs. standard treatment in the management of diabetic foot ulcers. Arch Surg 2002;137(7):822–7.

[12] Rosenberg L, De la Torre J. Wound healing, growth factors; phases of wound healing. eMedicine Plastic Surg 2006;457:3–6.

[13] Mercandetti M, Cohen AJ. Wound healing, healing and repair; sequence of events in wound healing. eMedicine Plastic Surg 2005;411:5–7.

[14] Reuterdahl C, Sundberg C, Rubin K, et al. Tissue localization of beta receptors for platelet-derived growth factor and platelet-derived growth factor B chain during wound repair in humans. J Clin Invest 1993;91(5):2065–75.

[15] Battegay EJ, Rupp J, Iruela-Arisepa L, et al. PDGF-BB modulates endothelial proliferation and angiogenesis in vitro via PDGF beta receptors. J Cell Biol 1994;125:917–28.

[16] Bar RS, Boes M, Booth BA, et al. The effects of platelet-derived growth factor in cultured microvessel endothelial cells. Endocrinology 1989;124:1841–8.

[17] Thommen R, Humar R, Misevic G, et al. PDGF-BB increases endothelial migration on cord movements during angiogenesis in vitro. J Cell Biochem 1997;64:403–13.

[18] Reinmuth N, Liu W, Jung YD, et al. Induction of VEGF in perivascular cells defines a potential paracrine mechanism for endothelial cell survival. FASEB J 2001;15(7):1239–41.

[19] Sato Y, Hamanaka R, Ono J, et al. The stimulatory effect of PDGF on vascular smooth muscle cell migration is mediated by the induction of endogenous basic FGF. Biochem Biophys Res Commun 1991;174(3):1260–6.

[20] Cao R, Brakenheilm P, Pawliuk R, et al. Angiogenic synergism, vascular stability and improvement of hind-limb ischemia by a combination of PDGF-BB and FGF-2. Nat Med 2003;5(9):604–13.

[21] Folkman J, D'Amore PA. Blood vessel formation: what is its molecular basis? Cell 1996;87(7):1153–5.

[22] Hirschi KK, Rohovsky SA, Beck LH, et al. Endothelial cells modulate the proliferation of mural cells precursors via platelet-derived growth factor-BB and heterotypic cell contact. Circ Res 1999;84:298–305.

[23] Benjamin LE, Hemo I, Keshet E. A plasticity window for blood vessel remodeling is defined by pericyte coverage of the preformed endothelial network and is regulated by PDGF-B and VEGF. Development 1998;125:1591–8.

[24] Korff T, Kimmina S, Martiny-Baron G, et al. Blood vessel maturation in a 3-dimensional spheroidal co-culture model: direct contact with smooth muscle cells regulates endothelial cell quiescence and abrogates VEGF responsiveness. FASEB J 2001;15:447–57.

[25] Doxey DL, Ng MC, Dill RE, et al. Platelet-derived growth factor levels in wounds of diabetic rats. Life Sci 1995;57:1111–23.

[26] Hammond HK, McKirnan MD. Angiogenic gene therapy for heart disease: a review of animal studies and clinical trials. Cardiovasc Res 2001;49:561–7.

[27] Zhu W-H, Guo X, Villaschi S, et al. Regulation of vascular growth and regression by matrix metalloproteinase in the rat aorta model of angiogenesis. Lab Invest 2000;80(4):545–55.

[28] Smiell JM, Wieman TJ, Steed DL, et al. Efficacy and safety of becaplermin (recombinant human platelet-derived growth factor-BB) in patients with nonhealing, lower extremity diabetic ulcers: a combined analysis of four randomized studies. Wound Repair Regen 1999;7:335–46.

[29] Cullen B, Smith R, McCulloch E, et al. Mechanism of action of PROMOGRAN, a protease modulation matrix, for the treatment of diabetic foot ulcers. Wound Repair Regen 2002;10: 16–25.

[30] Ovington L, Cullen B. Matrix metalloprotease modulation and growth factor protection. WOUNDS 2002;14(Suppl 5):2–13.

[31] Steed DL, Donohoe D, Webster MW, Lindsley L , the Diabetic Ulcer Study Group. Effect of extensive debridement and treatment on the healing of diabetic foot ulcers. J Am Coll Surg 1996;183:61–4.

ELSEVIER
SAUNDERS

NURSING
CLINICS
OF NORTH AMERICA

Nurs Clin N Am 42 (2007) 467–484

Psoriasis: Hope for the Future

Mary Sullivan-Whalen, RN, MSN, FNP,
Patricia Gilleaudeau, RN, MSN, FNP*

*The Rockefeller University, Laboratory of Investigative Dermatology,
1230 York Avenue, New York, NY 10021, USA*

The "heartbreak of psoriasis," once an advertisement for shampoo directed at scaly scalps, is a reality that affects millions of people each day. Often, when one thinks of psoriasis, it is scaly patches on the knees and elbows that come to mind. For many sufferers of psoriasis, the extent is far greater, affecting not only their skin and possibly joints, but relationships, livelihoods, and psyches.

Psoriasis is a common, chronic skin disease affecting more than 2.6% of the United States population, although the disease has been present since at least early biblical times when it was first identified and written about by Hippocrates [1]. Approximately 7 million people have been diagnosed with the disease and many more remain undiagnosed or undertreated. This noncontagious disease seems to have a genetic link, often found in families over generations. Although it can occur at any age from infancy to geriatrics, it is often diagnosed between the ages of 15 and 35 years, with both genders and all races equally affected. Diagnosis is often determined by visual examination, although a skin biopsy offers the most definitive diagnosis.

Psoriasis is a very real skin disease that is also a disease of perception, not only on the part of the patient, but also by the health care provider and the public. The patient perceives the disease, not only by the percent of body surface area (BSA) involved, but also by how their life has been affected. Patients may present with reports of the disease being all over their body, although examination finds only a small percentage scattered across the surface. Lesions on the hands and lower arms may not be a problem for

This article is based on interactions with patients during various research studies supported by NIH grant numbers GCRC # MO1RR00102-42, CCTS # 1UL1RR024143-01, and K12 # 1KL2RR0244142-01.

* Corresponding author.

E-mail address: gilleap@rockefeller.edu (P. Gilleaudeau).

some patients, but be quite significant for a person who uses their hands in business, such as a typist or a waiter. One of the patients examined, when asked to describe the extent and severity of his disease, reported it to be mild, affecting only 20% of BSA. In actuality, the patient was diagnosed with very severe disease that covered approximately 80% of BSA.

Although it takes a great inner strength to deal with a disease that is both personal and public, it is often the reaction by others to psoriasis that causes the greatest impact on the patient's psyche. During the time of Hippocrates, individuals with psoriasis were treated as those with leprosy and were banned from the general population. On some levels, treatment of present-time psoriasis patients offers many similarities to that of biblical lepers. Although it has been proved that these skin eruptions are not contagious, individuals are fired daily because their skin is seen as disturbing to others. Family life is altered because a wave of the arm or the removal of clothing at the end of the day usually causes a cloud of scaly skin to be released. Imagine a father who enjoys the ocean and pool with his family, but now only attends if he can be completely covered. Psoriatic patients often awaken to bloody and scaly bedclothes, despite being unaware that they scratched their skin during the night. This can be disturbing to the patient and the partner, and some relationships are unable to withstand the altered body presentation.

Many patients encounter health care professionals who have limited knowledge of the disease and may be unaware of the appropriate treatments currently on the market. Many believe that the only treatment available is through the use of topical steroids, which may be inappropriate for the patient whose disease covers more than 10% of BSA, and whose health insurance may only provide a single 30-g tube of drug every month. Providers must be comfortable prescribing the current therapies available, and if not, they should refer patients to the appropriate resources.

It is now known and widely accepted that psoriasis is a disease of the immune system, mediated by the T lymphocyte of the skin. It is recognized as the most prevalent T cell–mediated inflammatory disease in adults [2]. The resulting skin is thick and scaly, often on a background of erythema. Normal activities of daily living are often difficult to perform because of this condition, and manual work becomes virtually impossible because of psoriatic arthritis. Nonsteroidal anti-inflammatory drugs and cyclooxygenase-2 inhibitors offer some relief, although they do not target the causative mechanisms of this arthritis, from which approximately 20% of psoriasis patients suffer [1].

Current research now focuses on impacting the immune system of the skin and not global (total) immunosuppression. The hope is that newly introduced medications will provide remissions, be easier to administer, have improved safety profiles, and be well tolerated with few side effects. Various therapies currently used are presented later in the discussion.

Disease description

Clinical appearance

There are several different types of psoriasis. The most common type is known as "psoriasis vulgaris" or "plaque-type psoriasis," which comprises 85% to 90% of patients. The features of this type are scaling, erythema, and induration. Lesions are often large discrete plaques. The intensity of these features varies from mild to very severe and is often influenced by where on the body they occur. The lesions often occur at sites of trauma or sites of scarring, usually elbows and knees, and are often symmetrical [3]. The other classic sites of involvement are the scalp, face, soles and palms, genitals, and intertriginous folds. Various degrees of nail involvement may be seen including pitting, onycholysis, and subungual hyperkeratosis. A moderate degree of scaling within the ear canal is common. In severe cases this may produce an impaction of scale within the ear canal causing hearing impairment. The extent of involvement can range from discrete, localized areas to generalized body involvement.

Other, less common types of psoriasis include guttate psoriasis (characterized by small teardrop-shaped lesions); inverse psoriasis (occurring in the axilla, genital creases, and intertriginous folds); and palmoplantar psoriasis (occurring on palms and soles) [4]. Two other rare types of psoriasis are erythrodermic psoriasis, characterized by total body redness with the absence of discrete plaques, and pustular psoriasis, characterized by sterile pustules that may occur on a small percentage of the body, although a more widespread form, called von Zumbusch's, may occur over most of BSA. Erythrodermic and pustular psoriasis are severe inflammatory forms of the disease, causing these patients to seem quite ill with systemic symptoms, such as shaking chills, fever, and high white blood count. These patients can appear as if they have sepsis. The danger in sending these patients to the emergency room for sepsis evaluation is that the septic work-up itself (numerous venipunctures including blood cultures, lumbar puncture, and so forth) can make these patients septic. This occurs when bacteria (most often staphylococci) that are present on their skin are introduced into their bloodstream.

In addition to skin lesions, psoriasis can attack the joints causing psoriatic arthritis. The same inflammatory changes that affect the skin, namely T-cell proliferation, can affect the joints. Among the most common joints affected are the hands and feet (distal interphalangeal joints) and the spine. Virtually any joint of the body can be affected, producing a wide variety of arthritic changes and joint deformity. Psoriatic arthritis can destroy joints, similar to rheumatoid arthritis.

Pathogenesis

Before the mid-1980s, psoriasis was predominately thought of as a disease caused by abnormal keratinocyte growth and development. It was assumed that keratinocyte hyperproliferation associated with abnormal keratinocyte differentiation was the primary cause of psoriasis. Research beginning in the mid-1980s implicated T cells, planting the seed that psoriasis might be an immune disease. The observation that psoriasis improved with the use of cyclosporine A (CSA) in transplant patients helped develop this hypothesis. In the early 1990s, an experiment was done using a targeted immune modifier, a fusion protein comprised of human interleukin-2 and fragments of diphtheria toxin ($DAB_{389}IL$-2), which selectively blocks the growth of activated lymphocytes but not keratinocytes, to treat psoriasis. The reversal of several molecular markers of epidermal dysfunction was associated with a marked reduction in intraepidermal $CD3^{+}$ and $CD8^{+}$ T cells, suggesting a primary immunologic basis for this widespread disorder [4]. It is now recognized that epidermal hyperplasia is a reaction to the activation of the immune system in focal skin regions, which in turn is mediated by $CD8^{+}$ and $CD4^{+}$ T lymphocytes that accumulate in diseased skin. In contrast to uninvolved skin, T cells are dramatically increased in both the epidermis and dermis [5]. Other examples of T cell–mediated diseases are Crohn's disease, rheumatoid arthritis, multiple sclerosis, and juvenile-onset diabetes.

The psoriatic cascade probably begins when specialized antigen-presenting cells known as "Langerhans cells" or "dermal dendritic cells" process antigens in the skin and migrate to the skin-draining lymph nodes. There, the antigen-presenting cells present the antigen to naive $CD45RA^{+}$ T cells and activate them, initiating their transformation into memory-effector $CD45RO^{+}$ T cells and subsequent clonal expansion. Activated memory-effector $CD45RO^{+}$ T cells then emigrate from the lymph nodes and migrate to the blood [6,7]. Still unknown is the skin-cell antigen or autoantigen that initiates this cascade [3]. Antigen-specific, memory-effector $CD45RO^{+}$ T cells migrate from blood vessels to the skin [7]. It is here that these T cells are activated by antigen-presenting cells presenting the same antigen, triggering a vigorous release of cytokines and chemokines [3,7]. Antigen-presenting cells activate T cells by bridging ICAM-1 and CD11a, along with costimulatory molecules, such as LFA-3, CD40, and B7, causing an immunologic synapse to form. The T cell in turn emits cytokines and chemokines that expand the inflammatory infiltrate and stimulate the hyperproliferation of keratinocytes, resulting in clinical symptoms [3,7]. Examples of several important cytokines and chemokines are interferon-γ and tumor necrosis factor-α, which are secreted by T cell and directly induce keratinocyte production of inflammatory proteins, although other more complex inflammatory responses are also triggered.

Histologic features

Histologically, psoriasis is characterized by (1) thickening of the epidermis with rete elongation, keratinocyte hyperplasia, and incomplete terminal differentiation of keratinocytes (parakeratosis); (2) infiltration of skin

lesions by leukocytes; and (3) vascular elongation (angiogenesis) and dilata-
tion [5]. Other defining features include the presence of neutrophils within
small foci in the stratum corneum and significant mononuclear infiltrates
in the epidermis, which are detectable with immunostaining.

Description of disease as related by psoriasis patients

Imagine having a patient with poison ivy. In poison ivy, the patient experiences intense pruritus, which is exacerbated and bleeds the more the rash is
scratched. There are medicines available to help with the pruritus including
creams, ointments, and gels, but these can be messy. There are also systemic
antihistamines, but these can cause drowsiness. Still, the patient does not
fear because the cause of poison ivy is known, and can be avoided in the
future. Psoriasis, however, is a chronic disease. It is frequently accompanied
by pruritus and unlike poison ivy, its symptoms are not often relieved.
Although exacerbations and remissions may be experienced by some,
most people live with it on a daily basis. The cause or trigger is unknown.
Because the cause is unknown, its occurrence cannot be prevented. The
exact inheritance pattern is unknown, because not all people have family
links to the disease. Psoriasis causes functional impairments. Many patients
lose their jobs because of their illness, either because they cannot physically
do their job, or are discriminated against. Patients have difficulty walking,
climbing, or grasping objects because of psoriasis on their soles or palms.
They have restricted bending or crouching because the psoriasis over mov-
ing joints cracks and bleeds. There are limitations on stretching because the
skin splits or tears. Patients are unable to wear required tool belts or business attire that exacerbates psoriasis plaques on the trunk. They may be unable to sit because of psoriasis on the buttocks. Erythrodermic psoriasis may
cause chills and fever, which create difficulty controlling body temperature.
Psoriatic arthritis can disable various joints. Life-threatening systemic
infections or complications of cardiac and pulmonary systems caused by
erythrodermic and generalized pustular psoriasis may occur.

Beyond the physical symptoms are the insults to the quality of life. It is
not uncommon for patients to complain of chronic sleep deprivation from
severe pruritus, and depression related to perceived disfigurement and social
rejection. The authors have seen a dentist lose his business and a waiter lose
his job because of psoriasis on the hands, and have seen a teenage boy quit
school and become a hermit in his own home because he was so ashamed of
his appearance. Patients are ashamed to disrobe and have intimate relationships. One author (PG) used to say that psoriasis was not life threatening,
until she was corrected by a patient. He said that psoriasis often made
him feel like committing suicide.

Discrimination not only is seen in the general population, but from health
care professionals who themselves have limited understanding of the disease.
Patients may not have been treated by their health care provider as someone

having a treatable illness. They may have not been offered realistic treatment ("You have a chronic disease, you'll have to live with it.") These patients may be mistrustful of health care providers. Practitioners may need to earn their trust before treatment. To illustrate, here are some quotes from patients:

- "He (the doctor) told me nothing could be done."
- "He gave me a small tube of ointment and told me to return in 6 weeks." (This patient had 85% of his body affected)
- "I have been using this ointment all over my body continuously for 9 months." (Temovate ointment)
- "I keep telling the doctor that this ointment is not working."
- "I was told that anything other than creams and ointments can kill me." (This patient was asking about alternatives because topicals were not working)
- "I have been getting the same dose for 2 months." (UVB treatment)

Therapeutic options

Treatment can be divided into the following classifications: topical therapies, ultraviolet light therapy, systemic therapies, or biologic therapies.

Topical treatment

Steroids

Steroids are divided into classes by the strength or potency, from mild to very high potency. Often prepared as an ointment, cream, foam, or drops, it is applied directly to the lesions, usually on a daily or twice daily regimen. Topicals should be prescribed for the patient with limited disease, occurring on surface areas easily accessible by the patient. Depending on the involved areas, the preparation is chosen that is best applied to the specific area. Scalp preparations are best used when applied to wet hair and may require overnight application with morning rinse. Others may be applied directly to scalp and the hair then dried with removal of the product not required. It is not uncommon for steroids to be prescribed in the high or very high potency categories as first-time, first-line therapy. Although the patient may note improvement fairly quickly, they may also experience tachyphylaxis or the drug soon ceasing to work. Rebound may also be seen when the drug is overused and abused, and the resulting lesions may prove very difficult to treat and response may be either slow or absent [1,8]. The authors find in their practice that in using topical steroids it is best to start low and go slow.

Patient preference and the impact a preparation type has on the patient's garments, such as ointments, helps to drive the decision. Some patients prefer to use a cream during the day under work clothes and ointments at night before bedtime. Medication should only be applied to affected skin and every effort made to avoid nonlesional surfaces, which may be difficult depending on the proximity of the lesions.

Steroids should be considered for short or transient therapy, because they can produce many undesirable side effects. Long-term application of steroids has the potential to cause stretch marks to the area and may cause significant thinning of the skin because of degradation of collagen. Because of this specific effect, only low-potency steroids, such as over-the-counter hydrocortisone 1%, should be used for the face and genitals.

A more severe effect can occur with long-term use (years) of mid- to high-potency steroids. Absorption of the medication is a real risk that should be considered, with potentially life-threatening consequences, with a resulting adrenal insufficiency [8].

Potential therapies may unfortunately be dictated by health insurance plans held by the patient. It is not uncommon to find only selected drugs on formularies and there is often a limitation on the amount of drug dispensed, presenting a problem to the patient with significant disease and limited resources.

Vitamin D analogues

Vitamin D analogues serve to inhibit keritinocyte proliferation and induce terminal differentiation of psoriatic cells [1,2]. Often applied once to twice daily, they have been used successfully in combination with topical steroids. Although local irritation can occur early in therapy, they are well tolerated by the general population. Treatment should be limited to affected areas and time because of potential affects on calcium-phosphate homeostasis [1,2]. Patients should be aware that positive response (clearance) to these medications is often slow, but that continued and consistent use of the medication can prove rewarding and long lasting.

A combination drug of a vitamin D analogue and a topical steroid, known as Taclonex, has been approved by the US Food and Drug Administration (FDA) and is available at local pharmacies.

Ultraviolet light therapy

Psoralen plus UVA

The use of systemic psoralen plus UVA (PUVA) was considered one of the standards of psoriatic therapy until the 1990s. Treatment consisted of either the ingestion or bath with psoralen, a photosensitizing agent administered to the patient, and followed by UVA light therapy. The increased dosing of light facilitates clearance. Side effects may include burning but it may be more delayed than the burn seen post-UVB therapy, often not seen until 24 to 48 hours post therapy [1,9]. Patients may also complain of gastrointestinal disturbances, dizziness, and headache and may find that their eyes are more sensitive to light, necessitating the use of eye protection when venturing outdoors.

Clearance was seen in most patients, although the duration of clearance is variable and patient specific. Unfortunately, while performing a dermatologic examination on a patient many years post-PUVA, these patients have a notable freckling of the skin, representative of skin damage, and require extensive skin screening to rule out potential carcinoma of the skin. PUVA has been linked to the development of melanoma and patients require more frequent skin screening and skin mapping.

As safer and more conclusive therapies have been developed, PUVA as a therapy has fallen out of favor, but may prove beneficial in the older patient who has proved recalcitrant to other therapies, or for the patient with prior or current medical conditions that preclude treatment with other standard therapies, such as cancer and HIV.

PUVA used in combination with acitretin has proved successful in the patient suffering with either erythrodermic or pustular psoriasis. Caution should be used in the timing of the commencement of acitretin. Administration should be started 2 weeks before beginning PUVA or at the same time, to prevent photosensitization or burning. If it is decided to start acitretin after the start of PUVA, dosing of light should be decreased to prevent the potential for burning [1,9].

Broadband UVB

A popular form of light therapy, broadband UVB continues to be used in multiple centers and practitioner offices across the country, particularly for the treatment of guttate and plaque psoriasis. Broadband is a range of wavelengths of light in the UVB light spectrum, and is used to treat psoriatic skin lesions. Although burning is possible as with other light therapies, careful monitoring of skin response and assurance that the patient understands what may be symptoms of burning are essential. Although erythema is the most notable as a sign of burning, excessive pruritus should also be considered as a sign of burning. Patients must be aware that for light therapy to act at its best, several activities should precede stepping into the light box. Protection for the eyes is essential to preventing damage and is best achieved with the use of goggles and cotton placed in the wells of the eye protection. At the authors' institution, a brown paper bag is placed over the head, which offers adequate protection to the face, where the skin is often delicate and more likely to be damaged. If psoriasis is present on the face, very short periods of light can be administered, although it rarely lasts more than several seconds.

Men are asked to wear an athletic supporter as a protective device for the genitals. Patients using this garment are asked to be very careful in the positioning of the supporter, so that previously unexposed skin does not suffer burning. Women may place a thin film of zinc oxide over their nipples to prevent irritation and exposure to light. Patients are asked to place their arms and hands in a comfortable position and to repeat this same placement at each session. Additionally, it is requisite that all scaly patches be covered with an oil-base product, such as mineral oil or baby oil. This activity is necessary because scale is opaque, and as such prevents the passage of light to the base of the lesions [1]. The presence of oil on scaly lesions causes the scale to become translucent, allowing the light to pass through to the lesions, and prompting healing of the psoriasis.

Broadband UVB may be used as monotherapy, or in conjunction with the use of topical steroids, vitamin D analogues, or anthralin. If topicals are used, they should be put on the psoriatic lesions after the light therapy session is complete [1].

Narrowband UVB

First studied in Europe, narrowband UVB was introduced to the United States in the mid 1990s. Narrowband (312 nm) UVB has been proved to be a highly effective therapy in the psoriasis arsenal. Maximal clearance is seen when light therapy is administered three sessions a week at increasing dosing of light. This has been a useful therapy and a viable option for many patients when other therapies are prohibited, possibly because of prior medical conditions. Although well tolerated, therapy is time consuming, but can be continued as a maintenance therapy for long-term treatment.

As with PUVA, burning may occur but can be minimized by determining the safe dosing before commencing therapy and carefully monitoring the patient's response to light. Basal cell carcinoma and squamous cell carcinoma (but not melanoma) may develop with the use of narrowband UVB, requiring frequent skin monitoring.

Goeckerman therapy

Goeckerman light therapy was the most popular therapy from the 1970s to 1990s, and was considered at that time the only viable treatment for psoriasis. Goeckerman therapy is a combination of UVB light therapy, narrowband or broadband UVB, together with the application of coal or wood tar in a petrolatum base [10]. Light therapy is done on a daily basis, followed by tar placed on the skin and maintained on the skin for 20 hours or more. To achieve positive results, patients were often treated on inpatient units and often committed to month-long stays in the hospital unit.

As other psoriasis therapies have been introduced, Goeckerman therapy has fallen out of favor. Many people find it difficult to commit to such a long stay, particularly when length clearance cannot be ensured. Day treatment centers continue to use this therapy as daily treatments with patients removing the tar preparation before returning home, at the end of the day.

Systemic therapy

Commonly, systemic therapy is offered to patients with severe, active psoriatic disease or when individuals experience rapid flares of the disease. All these medications, with the exception of acitretin, are immunosuppressive drugs. Attempts to modulate the immune system bring the potential for immediate or serious consequences. Research has shown that when the immune system is dampened, the theoretical risk for increased incidence of infection and the development of cancer is a very real concern. Before commencing treatment with any of these agents, patients should be medically cleared to participate in therapy and closely followed thereafter. The development of infection should be treated immediately and cancer screening, age-specific to the patient, should be diligently followed.

Methotrexate

Initially used as formidable chemotherapy, methotrexate (MTX) was found to be a useful therapy in the treatment psoriasis as early as the 1950s. Known as a global immunosuppressant, the entire body is affected by the drug. It was found to be most beneficial in the treatment of pustular psoriasis and severe psoriatic arthritis. MTX was thought to act on the rapidly dividing basal keratinocytes of psoriatic lesions. Additional research has shown that MTX induces apoptosis (cell death) in active T cells and keratinocytes [1,11]. When prescribed for plaque psoriasis, the addition of topical steroids is often beneficial to achieve clearance.

MTX is prescribed in doses of 5 to 25 mg weekly, and administered in divided doses every 12 hours over 36 hours or three doses. Although MTX may be administered orally, intramuscularly, and intravenously, the oral route is preferred for the psoriatic patient. Monitoring complete blood counts and liver function tests is a key to ensuring the safety of the patient receiving the medication. Calculation of cumulative dose is important as a guide to consider further safety testing. The American Academy of Dermatology has developed guidelines for monitoring hepatotoxicity. In patients without risk factors for liver damage, first liver biopsy should be performed after cumulative dose of 1 to 1.5 g MTX. Provided no significant abnormalities are found, liver biopsy should be repeated after each additional 1.5 g. When cumulative dose is greater than 4 g, biopsy should be performed after each additional 1 g. In patients with risk factors for liver damage, liver biopsy should be performed with 2 to 4 months of starting MTX and after each additional 0.5 to 1 g thereafter [12].

Common side effects experienced include nausea, anorexia, fatigue, headache, and alopecia. Leukopenia, thrombocytopenia, and further dysfunction of the bone marrow are among serious adverse events, necessitating discontinuation of the medication and further treatment for the resulting blood dyscrasias. Leucovorin is the treatment of choice to reverse the damage caused by the overdosing of MTX [1,11].

MTX should be avoided in the patient with known kidney dysfunction, because of the potential for increased toxicity related to poor renal clearance [11]. Although rare, interstitial pneumonia has been diagnosed during and following MTX therapy, but is less often seen in the psoriatic patient as compared with patients using the treatment for rheumatoid arthritis.

Patients with a known alcohol abuse history or using concomitant hepato-toxic drugs should also avoid MTX because of the increased incidence of hepatotoxicity [6].

Cyclosporine (Neoral)

Initially used as the primary medication to prevent rejection in the organ transplant patient, CSA was considered as a psoriatic therapy when it was noted that transplant patients afflicted with psoriasis showed clearance when treated with the drug. In psoriasis, CSA inhibits the antigen-present-ing capacity of the Langerhans cells and mast cell functions, such as degran-ulation and cytokine production [1,13].

CSA has been found to be effective in approximately 70% of patients treated for severe plaque, pustular, and erythrodermic psoriasis. Improve-ment in the skin is noted to occur fairly quickly, with nail improvement following close behind. Dosing for psoriasis usually starts at 5 mg/kg/d, administered orally in divided doses twice a day. Patients are asked to be consistent in the manner that they ingest the CSA (with or without meals, and taken at approximately the same time of day). Dosing regimen may vary from the consistent use of the medication for up to a year, as approved by the FDA, or pulse or intermittent therapy, which allows for drug therapy for several weeks to months, followed by the discontinuation for the same time span, and then the restart of the medication [1,14].

Two potentially severe side effects, often dose related, that might occur while on the drug include hypertension and renal impairment. Close moni-toring of blood pressure and kidney function tests (blood urea nitrogen, creatinine), is imperative to ensure the health and safety of the patient. CSA has been shown also to raise total cholesterol and triglyceride levels [1,13]. Before commencing any therapy, the authors' dermatology research practice works closely with the patient's primary care provider to educate them as to potential negative effects that may necessitate prescribing additional treatment to address the adverse effects (ie, antihypertensive and cholesterol-lowering medications).

Severity of side effects has a direct correlation to the total daily CSA dose. Patients are instructed to drink two or more liters of liquids (water, juices, or carbonated beverages) each day to ensure kidney health. Before prescribing CSA, the practitioner should determine the patient's ability to understand safety issues and potential problems that may arise. The patient should not have a lifestyle that precludes them from drinking large amounts of water, such as a train conductor or a construction worker (both may have limited access to a bathroom), presenting possibly serious safety issues. If patients are either unable or unwilling to comply with these instructions and kidney function tests show impairment, namely a creatinine rise of 30% from baseline measurements, the medication should be either weaned to a safer level or discontinued immediately [1,13]. To avoid these potential problems, patients should begin a tapering of the CSA as soon as possible.

Fast tapers should be avoided because abrupt cessation of the medication may contribute to flaring of psoriasis. This may prove difficult to control and contribute to a dilemma, because the medication to control and treat flares is CSA.

Planning for additional treatment post-CSA should be addressed as soon as the patient starts therapy. Light therapy is both a viable and safe option post-CSA, and should commence while the patient is being slowly weaned. Planning and implementing a plan helps to ensure that a severe flare is not devastating.

Acitretin (Soriatane)

Acitretin is a derivative of vitamin A, a member of a class of drugs known as "retinoids." Acitretin regulates the excessive growth of keratinocytes, calming the hyperproliferation of cells. It seems to have some anti-inflammatory effects by inhibiting neutrophil function [1,15].

Because of its short half-life of 2 to 3 days, acitretin is a viable replacement for etretinate (an older vitamin A derivative), which because of its long half-life (>100 days) presents many serious health issues as it accumulate in the tissues. Research has shown that a portion of acitretin may be re-esterified in vivo into isoacitretin and etretinate [1,15]. Women of childbearing age should avoid this medication at all costs. If this is the only drug for the patient, precautions must be in place and understood by the patient to avoid pregnancy with the use of two methods of contraception [1,15].

It is common to prescribe acitretin in addition to light therapy (PUVA) for the treatment of plaque psoriasis. This combination is known as "RE-PUVA." Dosing of the medication is related to the severity of the disease.

Side effects seem to dose related. These include chelitis, sicca symptoms of the eyes and mouth, generalized pruritus, dry skin, loss of the stratum corneum of the soles and palms, alopecia, muscle and joint pain, and gastro-intestinal distress [1]. Serum lipid panels should be closely monitored, particularly in the patient with known lipid abnormalities. Acitretin should be used with caution in the patient with obesity, diabetes, smoking history, and alcohol abuse [1]. Liver enzymes should be monitored closely and dosing adjusted as required. The expected length of therapy is usually 3 to 4 months. Liver and kidney function tests, serum glucose, and lipid panels should initially be done every 3 weeks for several months, then every 2 months [1].

This is not a therapy to be considered if pregnancy is a possibility. Both men and women of childbearing age should use the medication with caution. In addition, pregnancy should be avoided up to 2 years after the discontinuation of therapy [1].

Biologic immunosuppressive therapy

This category includes four medications that have been approved by the FDA for the treatment on psoriasis. This new selection of drugs is seen to target the T cell in the skin and the various proteins and cytokines expressed, instead of globally suppressing the immune system, as many of the previously described drugs did. It must be remembered and recognized that any attempt to modulate the immune system brings with it the potential for immediate or serious consequences. Research has shown that when the immune system is dampened, the theoretical risk for increased incidence of infection and the development of cancer is a very real concern. Before commencing treatment with any of these agents, patients should be medically cleared to participate in therapy and closely followed thereafter. The development of infection should be treated immediately and cancer screening, age-specific to the patient, should be diligently followed.

Etanercept (Enbrel)

Enbrel was initially approved in the spring of 2002 for the treatment of rheumatoid and psoriatic arthritis. As research continued, psoriasis was also found to respond very positively to therapy. For the first time, not only was skin clearing, but arthritis also improved. Enbrel was FDA approved in April 2004 as first-line therapy in the treatment of psoriasis. Enbrel has been in the research pipeline since the early 1990s and has been used safely and tolerated in children with juvenile rheumatoid arthritis from the age of 4 years.

Enbrel is a biologic agent that targets and inhibits tumor necrosis factor, one of the culprits thought to contribute to psoriasis. Not only does it halt the progression of damage attributed to psoriatic arthritis, which is verified by serial radiologic examinations, but also significant skin response is seen in the first 3 months of therapy [16–18].

Dosing of Enbrel is 50 mg, subcutaneously injected by the patient, twice a week for 12 weeks, and then continued as long-term therapy with 50 mg dosed once a week. Although blood tests are not required, a pretreatment purified protein derivative (tuberculin) test is recommended, and repeated on a yearly basis or more frequently if the patient has known exposure to tuberculosis. Tumor necrosis factor inhibitors as a group have been connected with the reactivation of tuberculosis [16–18].

This medication has been fairly well tolerated by patients with few complaints. The most notable side effect has been injection site reaction, which is usually of short duration (minutes to hours) before clearance occurs and has been seen to cause little disturbance in patients' lives. Headache has been reported and is usually treated with analgesics, such as acetaminophen or ibuprofen.

Patients are also thrilled with Enbrel because it provides an opportunity for a drug holiday. This is to say that once the medication is stopped, clearance that has been achieved may continue for several weeks to months, with return of psoriasis occurring slowly, allowing the patient to cease continual therapy as desired during the year.

Efalizumab (Raptiva)

Raptiva was FDA approved as primary therapy for psoriasis vulgaris in October 2003. Its mode of action is to break the chain of CD11a, halting the advance of psoriasis [16,18,19]. Unfortunately, this is not a permanent break in the chain and return of disease should be expected once treatment is stopped.

Raptiva is fairly well tolerated, although a small number of patients report mild flulike symptoms in the early weeks of therapy. These symptoms include headache, fatigue myalgia, and increased temperatures, and resolve with little or no medical intervention.

Long-term concerns include the development of thrombocytopenia, which can be both severe and acute in presentation. Treatment includes the discontinuation of Raptiva and the use of prednisone, tapered to the platelet response. Should this adverse event occur, it is wise to enlist the assistance of a hematologist to help provide direction in the treatment of the patient with thrombocytopenia. Safety monitoring for the patient on Raptiva includes serial complete blood counts, initially monthly for several months and continued with platelet surveillance every 2 to 3 months thereafter.

Another phenomenon that has occurred during treatment with Raptiva is with the introduction of new small psoriatic lesions, now known as "papules of Papp" or "Papp's papules." Occurring across the BSA, although they are not dangerous or foreboding, their appearance can be very disconcerting for patients who may view this as ultimately the return of disease despite being on psoriasis-specific therapy. In their practice, the authors have found that continued treatment with Raptiva rectifies the situation with the resolution of the papules. This occurrence should not be viewed by either the patient or the practitioner as a failure of therapy, but rather as an expected although uncommon side effect.

Should the patient on Raptiva decide to discontinue therapy, a follow-up plan should be in place. It is not uncommon for a flare of psoriasis to occur, with the return of disease presenting differently than the original presentation. Psoriasis may now be seen in areas where it had not been previously, with varying characteristics of erythema and scale. This return of disease can be devastating to the patient and rescue therapy should be implemented immediately with CSA.

Amevive (Alefacept)

The first drug to be FDA approved as a primary treatment for psoriasis was Amevive. Introduced in the spring of 2002, it was welcomed by both patients and practitioners alike. Amevive inhibits the production of LFA-1, and stops the production of CD2, halting the response of T cells [10,16].

Administered intramuscularly in a practitioner's office, it is dosed at a set rate of 15 mg and is administered for 12 weeks. Patients are required to stop the medication for the next 12 weeks and may restart another course soon after if needed. Clearance with Amevive is slow with maximal response noted at week 17. Although only approximately 25% of patients have significant response, it is interesting that of those who choose to attempt a second course of treatment, many experience a better response and clearance may often last weeks to months. It is well tolerated by most patients, although some do report mild flulike symptoms in the first 1 to 3 weeks of treatment.

Infliximab (Remicade)

The most recently approved FDA drug is Remicade. This is not meant to be prescribed as a first-line agent; rather, it is to be used for refractory disease. Previously approved for use in the treatment of rheumatoid arthritis and Crohn's disease, Remicade, a drug in the tumor necrosis factor inhibitor family, was shown as effective therapy for psoriasis. Administered as an infusion, it is dosed at 5 to 10 mg/kg per infusion on weeks 0, 2, and 6. Significant clearance of disease is noted in most patients. The response rate, extent, and rapidity of clearance with Remicade were similar to the response seen in CSA [16,18,20].

Many patients on therapy report an excellent outcome by week 10. As with Enbrel, patients should have purified protein derivative (tuberculin) tests placed before the start of therapy, and followed by yearly testing. Headache seems to be the most common side effect, although infusion reactions have also been seen.

Future research

Although substantial work has been done thus far, much more is needed. To date, many of the mechanistic studies, done at The Rockefeller University, have been the impetus to finding not only answers as to the potential cause of the disease but also to investigate and understand fully the actions of the current drugs used in the treatment of psoriasis. Unfortunately, no animal model of psoriasis exists, but these models have the potential to give understanding as to how complex inflammatory circuits are regulated [21]. Unfortunately, even though this research presents deficiencies, they serve to offer a jumping off point for future studies and the hope for many more questions to be answered.

One of the questions being tackled at the authors' center is whether psoriasis is an actual disease attributed to the overstimulation of the immune system, or are skin cells reacting to changes in the normal stimulation of the immune system [21]. Another troubling question yet to be answered is, how can one best determine, before commencing therapy with a known effective medication, which drug will produce the most favorable response for that specific patient and present fewer safety concerns.

Finally, clinicians must be ensured that despite multiple agents potentially used over extended periods, years, or decades, a patient's immune system remains intact without seeing potentially devastating disease caused by these treatments [21]. The work to answer these questions continues, and it is hoped that additional drugs are found that present with even better safety profiles, short and long term, and are well tolerated.

How to decide treatment

Treatment of psoriasis should be dictated by the extent of disease, the impact on the individual's activities of daily living, past medical history, and the patient's ability to participate in his or her therapy. Psoriasis is a very real skin disease that is also a disease of perception. When discussing therapy with a patient, health care providers need to listen to the patient's perception of themselves. This is very important and greatly influences what therapy is offered. Caregivers cannot possibly know how a person with psoriasis feels or thinks of their appearance. Someone with 80% of their body affected with severe plaques may not be bothered by their disease or appearance. Yet, he or she may not want to risk any systemic therapy. Another patient, however, with 5% of their body affected may be so disturbed by their disease that they may wish to embark on systemic therapy. It is the goal of health care providers to support the patient in deciding what treatment is best for them. If a health care provider proposes what they think is the ideal treatment, but the patient is terrified about potential side effects, this is obviously not the ideal treatment for this patient.

The authors suggest beginning as one would with any other patient. Take a complete history not only of their psoriasis, but of other medical problems and illness, past and present. Inquire what medications they take, including over-the-counter vitamins and supplements. Psoriasis patients try over-the-counter vitamins and supplements, sometimes at the suggestion of a concerned relative or friend. Something in their medical history or medicine list may exclude a certain therapeutic option. Do they drink alcohol? This necessitates caution with a hepatotoxic drug, such as MTX. Do they have a support system (family or friends)? How far do they live from the clinic? If a patient lives 3 hours away, phototherapy two or three times a week is difficult. Does the patient have health insurance? The authors are fortunate to work in a research setting, where patients receive free care and medicines. How do they feel (both physically and emotionally)? A claustrophobic patient may not be able to stand in a light box. A patient with severely arthritic hands may not be able to handle giving themselves an injection. Assess what a patient knows about their disease; do not assume. Use this visit to educate. The bottom line is to get to know the patient. Take cues not only from what the patient says but also what he or she does not say. Body language speaks volumes.

The next step is to assess the psoriasis. Have them take off their clothes. One author (PG) found a suspicious lesion on an elderly man that turned out to be a melanoma. The patient said it had been there for several years, but he had never shown it to his dermatologist because he had never been asked to disrobe. When examining the patient, it is important to touch the skin. Remember, these patients may have been treated as if they had a contagious disease. This myth needs to be dispelled. The authors try to touch patients at every visit (shake their hand, feel their skin, hug them, and so forth).

After doing a thorough skin examination, consider patient comfort and allow the patient to get dressed before discussing treatment options. Outline appropriate therapies available and clearly delineate advantages and disadvantages for each therapy and encourage the patient to do the same. Be realistic and honest. A psoriasis patient needs to become part of the team in regard to deciding and receiving therapy. The authors always err on the safe side when suggesting therapy, again taking cues not only from what the patient says but also from what he or she does not say. Encourage the patient to involve their support system when making a decision regarding therapy. Encourage the family to ask questions, either at a visit or by telephone, and invite them to be part of the team. Encourage patients to learn as much as possible about their disease and treatment options. This allows them to act as their own advocate and take an active role in care decisions. Patients should know that they are not alone; resources are available, such as The National Psoriasis Foundation (www.psoriasis.org or 800-723-9166). Together with patients, clinicians strive to improve their lives and offer hope for the future.

Summary

Psoriasis is a chronic disease that affects almost 3% of the population, yet many health care professionals do not know much about the disease. This leads to patient frustration, caused by not being offered adequate treatment, and provider frustration, caused by the lack of knowledge regarding therapeutic options. It is hoped that the information conveyed in this article provides insight regarding how to make the diagnosis and potential therapeutic options. Great strides have been made in knowing what happens on the cellular level. This has led to the development of more therapeutic options for psoriasis. Providers need to work with the patient and arrive at a decision together for therapy that is appropriate, that all parties are comfortable with, and that does not cause dangerous side effects. The key to this is education on the part of the provider and the patient.

Acknowledgments

The authors thank James G. Krueger, our collaborating physician, for his tireless support and contribution to our knowledge base; colleagues in the Laboratory of Investigative Dermatology for their support; the nursing staff at the Rockefeller University Hospital for their expert caring of our patients; and Geoffrey Gilleaudeau for help in editing this manuscript.

References

[1] Christophers E, Mroweitz U. Psoriasis. In: Freedberg IM, Eisen AZ, Wolff K, et al, editors. Fitzpatrick's dermatology in general medicine. 6th edition. New York: McGraw Hill; 2003. p. 407–27.

[2] Koo JYM, Siebenlist J. Vitamin D analogues in the treatment of psoriasis. In: Roenigk HII, Maibach HI, editors. Psoriasis, 3rd edition. New York: Marcel Dekker, Inc.; 1998. p. 497–510.

[3] Griffiths CEM, Clark CM, Chalmers RJG, et al. A systematic review of treatments for severe psoriasis. Health Technol Assess 2000;4(40):1–125.

[4] Drake LA, Ceilley RI, Cornelison RL, et al. Guidelines of care for psoriasis. J Am Acad Dermatol 1993;28(4):632–7.

[5] Gottlieb SL, Gilleaudeau P, Johnson R, et al. Response of psoriasis to a lymphocyte-selective toxin ($DAB_{389}IL-2$) suggests a primary immune, but not keratinocyte, pathogenic basis. Nat Med 1995;1(5):442–7.

[6] Wang F, Lew W, Krueger JG. The therapy of psoriasis based on innate and adaptive immune mechanisms of disease pathogenesis. G Ital Dermatol Venereol 2004;139(3):207–30.

[7] Grabbe S, Schwartz T. Immunoregulatory mechanisms involved in elicitation of allergic contact hypersensitivity. Immunol Today 1998;19:37–44.

[8] Amin S, Cornell RC, Stoughton RB, et al. Topical corticosteroids. In: Roenigk HH, Maibach HI, editors. Psoriasis. 3rd edition. New York: Marcel Dekker, Inc.; 1998. p. 453–67.

[9] Ortel B, Liebman EJ, Honigsmann H, et al. Oral psoralen photochemotherapy. In: Roenigk HH, Maibach HI, editors. Psoriasis. 3rd edition. New York: Marcel Dekker, Inc.; 1998. p. 543–57.

[10] Gibson LE, Perry HO. Goeckerman therapy. In: Roenigk HH, Maibach HI, editors. Psoriasis. 3rd edition. New York: Marcel Dekker, Inc.; 1998. p. 469–77.

[11] Roenigk HH, Maibach HI. Methotrexate. In: Roenigk HH, Maibach HI, editors. Psoriasis. 3rd edition. New York: Marcel Dekker, Inc.; 1998. p. 609–29.

[12] Chalmers RJG, Kirby B, Smith A, et al. Replacement of routine liver biopsy by procollagen III aminopeptide for monitoring patients with psoriasis receiving long-term methotrexate: a multicentre audit and health economic analysis. Br J Dermatol 2005;152:444–50.

[13] Koo JYM, Gambla C, Lee J. Cyclosporin for the treatment of psoriasis. In: Roenigk HH, Maibach HI, editors. Psoriasis. 3rd edition. New York: Marcel Dekker, Inc.; 1998. p. 641–58.

[14] Zachariae H. Long-term use of cyclosporine in dermatology. In: Roenigk HH, Maibach HI, editors. Psoriasis. 3rd edition. New York: Marcel Dekker, Inc.; 1998. p. 659–62.

[15] Goldfarb MT, Ellis C. Clinical use of etretinate and acitretin. In: Roenigk HH, Maibach HI, editors. Psoriasis. 3rd edition. New York: Marcel Dekker, Inc.; 1998. p. 663–70.

[16] Nussbaum R, Krueger JG. Treatment of inflammatory dermatoses with novel biologic agents: a primer. Adv Dermatol 2002;18:45–89.

[17] Available at: www.enbrel.com. Accessed December 1, 2006.

[18] Available at: www.psoriasis.org. Accessed December 1, 2006.

[19] Available at: www.raptiva.com. Accessed December 1, 2006.

[20] Available at: www.remicade.com. Accessed December 1, 2006.

[21] Lowes MA, Bowcock AM, Krueger JG. Pathogenesis and therapy of psoriasis. Nature 2006;44:866–73.

ELSEVIER
SAUNDERS

Nurs Clin N Am 42 (2007) 485–500

NURSING
CLINICS
OF NORTH AMERICA

Aging Skin: Causes, Treatments, and Prevention

Paula E. Bermann, MSN, RN, APRN, BC, DNC

303 East 48th Street, Savannah, GA 31405, USA

Aging is a complex process that results in functional and aesthetic changes in the skin. As advances in skin biology have broadened understanding of the aging process, new treatments have been developed and old treatments refined to retard aging and rejuvenate the skin. This article focuses on the mechanism of aging, including photoaging, cosmeceuticals used to combat the aging process, cosmetic procedures popular with an aging population, and a primary means of preventing the effects of photoaging: sunscreen.

Intrinsic and extrinsic aging

As individuals age, the skin undergoes changes such as irregular pigmentation, sallowness, and loss of elasticity. Biologic processes lead to a decrease in function and the ability to tolerate injury. Genetic and environmental processes contribute to the aging process.

Two general theories of aging support these decreases [1]. The first postulates that aging is a preordained process that is genetically determined. It states that, because chromosomes shorten at every cell cycle, apoptosis or planned cell destruction occurs at a predetermined interval. The second theory suggests that aging is caused by cumulative environmental damage, such as that caused by ultraviolet (UV) radiation and oxidation.

These theories may also be described as *intrinsic* and *extrinsic* processes. The intrinsic, or chronologic, component is regulated by genetic code and is usually combined with a defective repair system [2]. Although aging skin that has been protected from environmental assault may show laxity and thinning, it tends to retain its pigment and lacks actinic damage [3].

E-mail address: pebermann@aol.com

0029-6465/07/$ - see front matter © 2007 Elsevier Inc. All rights reserved.
doi:10.1016/j.cnur.2007.05.001

The extrinsic component is a cumulative process of degeneration induced by years of exposure to environmental toxins, such as solar UV light and cigarette smoke. Decades spent pursuing a healthy suntan are now shown to be a major cause of damage to the skin, also known as *photoaging*. In fact, photoaging is believed to be responsible for almost 80% of the skin changes commonly attributed to the aging process [4]. Normal skin maintains a dynamic collagen balance, which acts as the major structural protein in the skin. Fibroblasts produce new layers of collagen when collagen genes are activated. Recent research has discovered a complex genetic pathway through which UV radiation can reduce collagen synthesis and increase the destruction of collagen by shutting down the collagen-producing genes, while accelerating collagen destruction. This process produces tiny wounds, or microscars, that over a lifetime become macroscars, visible in the skin as wrinkles, irregular pigmentation, and a dry, leathery appearance. Sunlight accelerates the genetic destruction, whereas sun protection prevents this damaging process. In fact, the level of collagen production is completely back to normal within 2 days of stopping UV exposure [5].

Cosmeceuticals

Cosmeceuticals are agents present in many cosmetic products that provide physiologic benefits to the consumer. However, they are not considered true pharmaceuticals, because they do not necessarily show a biologic therapeutic benefit [6,7]. Cosmeceuticals are found in many forms, from antioxidants, to peptides, to skin lighteners and hydroxy acids. One area in which cosmeceuticals have delivered great benefit is the treatment of aging and photoaged skin.

Hydroxy acids

Many products have been promoted to address the skin's response to aging. Among some of the oldest are those that contain an alpha hydroxy acid (AHA). The skin-rejuvenating properties of these weak organic acids have been recognized for centuries. Cleopatra reportedly bathed in spoiled milk containing lactic acid and French noblewomen used spoiled wine containing tartaric acid to clean their faces [8].

Several different types of AHAs are found in nature. In addition to those mentioned earlier, many others have been used to address the effects of skin aging (Table 1). The most popular is glycolic acid, now produced synthetically in the laboratory. Since the early 1990s when glycolic acid products were first marketed, cosmetic companies have introduced hundreds of ways to apply AHAs to the skin. When applied topically, AHAs increase exfoliation and have a positive effect on the skin's ability to hold moisture [9]. Their exfoliative properties are the result of decreasing the cohesion of

Table 1
Commonly used alpha hydroxy acids and their sources

Type of acid	Source
Ascorbic	Fruits
Citric	Citrus fruits
Glycolic	Sugar cane
Lactic	Fermented milk products
Malic	Unripened apples
Mandelic acid	Bitter almonds
Oxalic	Sauerkraut, vegetables
Tartaric	Fermented grapes

cells in the *epidermis*, or outer layer of the skin, so that shedding of the outermost layers is facilitated. When these cells loosely adhere to the skin surface, as occurs in photoaging, the surface feels rough and scaly. Exfoliation provides immediate smoothing and a more uniform appearance. Depending on the concentration and pH of the AHA, this may include separating the epidermis from the dermis (epidermolysis), or *chemical peeling*. However, most AHAs are used in lower concentrations and thus simply accelerate cell loss and increase exfoliation.

The moisturizing effects of AHAs help diminish the appearance of fine wrinkles because these products help the epidermal layer retain water. These effects also help relieve rough, dry skin and maintain proper moisture content in healthy skin.

Another effect of these acids is increased epidermal thickness. In higher concentrations, such as those found in chemical peels, this includes the formation of new collagen in the dermis, which results in increased skin elasticity. AHAs also decrease uneven pigmentation and increase perfusion to the dermis, which is noticed as a radiant, youthful glow [10].

When selecting an AHA, choosing the proper vehicle is important. This vehicle helps determine the efficacy of the AHA and therefore should be chosen according to skin type and purpose of the product. Generally, creams are best for dry skin, lotions for combination skin, and alcohol-based or oil-free preparations for oily, acne-prone skin. Products may be formulated as facial creams and cleansers, astringents and toners, hand and body lotions, and shampoos and body cleansers. In many cases, the concentration of acid varies according to the type of product, with body lotions usually containing a higher acid concentration than products designed for the face.

Beta hydroxy acids (BHA) have long been used in over-the-counter (OTC) acne products. The most commonly used BHA is salicylic acid in concentrations from 2% to 12%. It acts primarily as a keratolytic but may be useful in enhancing the absorption of other products used for anti-aging, such as antioxidants. BHAs are an attractive alternative to AHAs for individuals who have sensitive skin or rosacea [11].

Finally, polyhydroxy acids are not a combination of the other hydroxy acids, as commonly believed, but are of a unique class. Gluconolactone is one of the most popular agents in this class and has been shown to have antioxidant properties, while sharing in some of the effects of AHAs, such as glycolic acid [12]. Several cosmetic manufacturers have incorporated polyhydroxy acids in their products. Among them is NeoStrata, which markets these products as gentler alternatives to their AHA line.

Retinol and retinoids

Vitamin A–based drugs, such as retinol, have been shown to reverse the signs of aging. Although it has a lower potency than the prescription retinoids, retinol can improve photodamage and stimulate the production of collagen with less irritation [13]. Prescription retinoids, such as tretinoin (Retin-A Micro, Renova, Ortho Neutrogena, Skillman, NJ) and tartrazine (Tazorac, Allergan, Inc., Irvine, CA), have long been a mainstay for preventing and treating photoaging [14]. The most commonly used drug in this group is tretinoin, which was first used to treat acne vulgaris. As early as 1983, researchers noted improvement in facial wrinkles in patients using it for acne, and since then many studies have shown that it is an effective treatment for the clinical effects of photoaging. Of these effects, the surface roughness, mottled hyperpigmentation, and fine wrinkles demonstrate the most significant improvement with tretinoin therapy [15]. This therapy works by increasing the capacity of the epidermis to hold water, resulting in a smoother feel and appearance. Tretinoin also increases collagen, which is essential in providing strength and resiliency, in the dermis, resulting in less sagging and thus a more youthful appearance. Furthermore, experts believe that it may also retard or prevent further damage as and before it occurs.

First marketed as Retin-A for acne, the product was reformulated with a less irritating, more emollient base and introduced as Renova, which was approved by the U.S. Food and Drug Administration (FDA) in 1996 for treating photodamaged skin. It is currently available as a solution or cream. A downside to tretinoin is its propensity to be irritating and the fact that the gains produced through daily use disappear when it is discontinued.

These retinoids are available through prescription only, but several other products containing vitamin A derivatives or retinol are available OTC. Although these products, usually labeled antiwrinkle or antiaging preparations, cannot produce the dramatic results obtained with tretinoin, many consumers are pleased with their cosmetic results.

Antioxidants

Some of the newest products for treating aging skin are those that contain antioxidants, such as vitamins C and E. Antioxidants are believed to protect the skin from photodamage through decreasing the ability of UV radiation to produce free radicals. Sunlight increases the production of these toxic molecules, which are missing an electron, hence the name *free radicals.* These cells search for a normal cell to donate an electron, which damages the normal cell. This damage is then noticed as the signs of aging mentioned earlier, or even as skin cancer. Antioxidants readily give up electrons to free radicals, thus enabling normal cells to remain intact. Vitamin C not only acts as an electron donor but also has been shown in the laboratory to repair collagen damage and stimulate its production [16]. It is also a very effective bleaching agent for skin lightening. Although available in several forms and concentrations, the most effective form has been shown to be L-ascorbic acid in a concentration exceeding 10%.

Another antioxidant, ferulic acid, has been combined with vitamins A and E to produce a more potent antioxidant effect than either agent used as monotherapy. Ferulic acid is present in the cell walls of grains, fruits, and vegetables. Its main function in preventing photoaging is its strong absorption of UV light, thus protecting skin from UV-induced erythema. A recent study found that adding ferulic acid to vitamins C and E not only stabilized the formulation but also doubled the photoprotection from four-fold to eightfold [17].

Alpha lipoic acid is an antioxidant and an anti-inflammatory agent that has been shown to interfere with the production of cytokines that produce inflammation [18]. It has also been shown to protect the naturally occurring antioxidants vitamins C and E in cells. Both clinical and objective measurements of photoaging have noted significant reduction in wrinkle measurement during treatment with alpha lipoic acid.

Coenzyme Q10 (CoQ10) is another antioxidant studied for its effect on aging skin. It is an important cell membrane nutrient and contributes to the ATP mitochondrial transport chain to produce energy within the cells [19]. Its name comes from the word *ubiquitous*, because it is found in every cell in the body. In vitro studies provide reasonable evidence supporting the use of CoQ10, but limited clinical data are available. As an antioxidant, it acts as a scavenger for free radicals.

Idebenone is similar in structure to CoQ10 but is believed to be stronger and more efficient than other well-known antioxidants, including alpha lipoic acid and vitamins C and E. Not only a potent free radical scavenger, idebenone also functions as an electron carrier and is effective under hypoxic conditions [20]. Idebenone has been used for more than 20 years outside the United States for treating neurologic disorders, such as Alzheimer's disease to enhance memory and repair defects in neurotransmission. It was recently formulated as a topical cream, containing 0.5% idebenone, and sold in department stores as Prevage MD (manufactured by agreement of Allergan and Elizabeth Arden by Allergan Inc., Irvine, CA). Like other antioxidants, it must be used consistently to prevent signs of aging.

Kinetin, or 0.1% N6-furfuryladenine, is a substance found in many yeast plants, where it functions as a plant growth regulator. In cell cultures, it has been shown to delay some critical biochemical and morphologic changes associated with aging. When added to fibroblasts, kinetin slowed changes in cell shape, growth rates, cell size, and molecular synthesis [21]. Investigators have surmised that the mechanism of action that results in age retardation may involve the genes that influence aging [5]. Some users have reported improvement in skin texture and reduction of mottled pigmentation. Increased photosensitivity with kinetin has not been reported. Several OTC cosmetics containing kinetin are currently on the market, including the Kinerase line by Valeant Pharmaceuticals (Aliso Viejo, CA).

Green tea is a powerful antioxidant, characterized by its topical anti-inflammatory effect, which is demonstrated by decreased white blood cell infiltrate and decreased edema from UVB after exposure. In addition, compounds found in green tea have been shown to influence biochemical pathways important in cell synthesis and responses of tumor promoters [22]. Green tea is believed to have antiaging effects through decreasing inflammation and acting as a scavenger for free radicals.

Investigators have recently measured the antioxidant capacity of many of the most popular antioxidants [23]. Agents such as idebenone, kinetin, CoQ10, alpha lipoic acid, and vitamin C were tested in vitro and in vivo for their effects on inhibiting UVB irradiation on human keratinocytes and products produced during oxidation were measured. The researchers reported that idebenone rated the highest in antioxidant capacity with a score of 95, followed by vitamin E (80), kinetin (68), CoQ10 (55), alpha lipoic acid (52), and vitamin C (52). Therefore, research supports the great potential of idebenone for preventing signs of aging.

Peptides/growth factors

The use of peptides is becoming more popular among consumers seeking effective treatments for aging and photoaging. Their main function is to control cell proliferation and differentiation and to stimulate the synthesis of collagen. Peptides also function as cellular communicators by providing instructions as to how specific cellular structures are intended to function. Much of what is known about peptides comes from the study of wound healing and studies in fetal skin that show the presence of growth factors, which result in scarless healing and a relative lack of inflammation [24]. This natural healing process is dependent on biologic factors that signal the start of the repair process. Macrophages secrete substances such as growth factors that begin a cascade of events leading to wound healing. Because skin aging is partially characterized by a decrease in collagen synthesis and an increase in collagen breakdown, biologic factors that stimulate collagen should slow or prevent this process.

Five key growth factors have been identified and are being studied for their effects on aging skin. The most important of these is transforming growth factor (TGF)-β, because most cell types have receptors for this peptide. TGF-β is a potent stimulator of collagen production and promotes synthesis of cell proteins [25]. In animals, it has been shown to accelerate wound healing after incision [26]. Currently available cosmeceuticals, including those from SkinMedica and Neocutis, contain single or multiple growth factors. Compared with other cosmeceuticals, products containing growth factors are expensive.

One of the newest peptides to be marketed for aging skin is KTTKS or matrixyl. This pentapeptide promotes collagen synthesis and increases the thickness of elastin fibers. Studies sponsored by the National Institutes of Health confirmed that KTTKS can promote the synthesis of collagen and fibronectin by cultured fibroblasts [27]. When palmitoyl (pal) was added to enhance penetration through the stratum corneum, pal-KTTKS was found to penetrate and remain in the dermis. Several products contain this peptide, including Olay Regenerist (Procter & Gamble, Cincinnati, OH) and Strivectin-SD (Klein-Becker USA, Salt Lake City, UT).

Copper peptides have been shown to increase fibroblast activity, which influences collagen and elastin synthesis and thus promotes skin repair. Copper acts as a carrier for cofactors needed for enzymatic steps in collagen production [28]. The development of products containing copper is based on evidence that it facilitates healing in diabetic foot ulcers and post–Mohs surgery by promoting vascular formation and synthesis of collagen and elastin. Its main advantage is that products containing copper peptides are inexpensive compared with other antioxidant preparations.

Skin lighteners and bleaching agents

Melasma is an irregular brown hyperpigmentation that often affects women and is usually found on the face and other sun-exposed areas. Although the precise cause of melasma is unknown, experts believe that genetic influences, exposure to UV radiation, pregnancy, hormonal therapies, cosmetics, or phototoxic drugs may be involved [29]. In the skin, melanocytes continuously produce melanosomes, which are distributed to the adjacent keratinocytes. This production cycle relies on the conversion of tyrosine to melanin through the enzyme tyrosinase. As with other diagnoses in which no cause is identified, many treatments for melasma are available. Current treatments include hypopigmenting agents, chemical peels, and lasers, sometimes used in combination.

The most commonly used hypopigmenting agent is hydroquinone, available OTC in a 2% concentration and by prescription as a 4% or higher strength. This agent is classified as a tyrosinase inhibitor, because it prevents the formation of melanin, thus preventing hyperpigmentation. Despite concerns over potential carcinogenesis seen in mouse studies, hydroquinone remains the most effective topically applied fading agent approved by the FDA for treatment of melasma [30]. It has recently been combined with topical steroids, glycolic acid, or tretinoin to increase its effectiveness.

Another agent shown to be somewhat effective in treating melasma is kojic acid. Derived from the fungus *Aspergillus oryzae*, it works by interfering with the production of melanocytes. Although classified as a tyrosinase inhibitor, pretreatment of mice with kojic acid before long-term UV exposure was found to decrease clinical assessments of wrinkling [31]. Kojic acid has a slightly increased chance of causing contact dermatitis [31].

Soy has also been used to decrease hyperpigmentation, but because of its estrogen-like effects on the skin, it may be deleterious in treating melasma [32]. However, it may be useful for treating other estrogen-related conditions, such as the skin thinning and collagen loss seen in postmenopausal women. Soy products can be found in the Aveeno skin care line from Johnson & Johnson Consumer Products Company (Skillman, NJ).

Soft tissue augmentation

Many other therapies are available for improving the structure and appearance of aging skin, including soft tissue augmentation, chemical peels, microdermabrasion, and laser resurfacing. Soft tissue augmentation involves the injection or insertion of a substance, or dermal filler, to smooth lines and wrinkles by providing support under the skin. These substances may be autologous, artificial, or heterologous, such as bovine collagen. Several injectable fillers are approved by the FDA for treating the subcutaneous atrophy (loss of fat) that accompanies aging. These products are used to augment soft tissue deficits by filling in the fine lines and sallowness resulting from photoaging and are also used for intrinsically aged skin. Some fillers are temporary and others permanent.

Some of the most popular fillers contain hyaluronic acid (HA), such as Restylane (Medicis Pharmaceutical Company, Scottsdale, AZ) and Juvederm (Allergan, Inc., Irvine, CA). When injected into and below the dermis, hyaluronic fillers combine with naturally occurring HA and bind to water. When applied topically, such as in the prescription emollient sodium hyaluronate (Hylira, Hawthorn Pharmaceuticals), it has been shown to increase water absorption and decrease transepidermal water loss, whereas when it is combined with diclofenac (Solaraze, Bradley Pharmaceticals, Inc, Fairfield, New Jersey) to treat actinic keratoses, it decreases irritation [33,34]. In the dermis, HA functions as a space-filling, cell-protective molecule that provides structure and volume and has a shock-absorbing role. It has been used as a surgical aid in eye surgery, as a supplement for joint fluid in arthritis, and to facilitate healing in surgical wounds [35]. During the aging process, the naturally occurring HA decreases, resulting in dermal dehydration and the formation of wrinkles. The addition of manufactured HA results in increased skin turgor and elasticity.

Today, HA gels are derived from animals and bacteria. A popular animal-based HA gel is Hylaform (Inamed Corporation, Santa Barbara, CA), which uses rooster combs as its source for the HA molecules. Several bacteria-derived HA fillers are on the market [36]. The most popular is Re-stylane (Medicis), which is produced through fermentation from cultured streptococcus bacteria. Captique (Inamed) and Juvederm (Allergan) are also non–animal-based HA fillers approved for treating moderate to severe facial wrinkles and folds around the face and mouth. Clinical effects from HA fillers can last from 4 to 6 months.

Another type of soft tissue filler contains poly-L-lactic acid (PLLA), which is a biodegradable, synthetic compound from the alpha hydroxy acid family. Manufactured by Dermik Laboratories (Berwyn, PA), Sculptra was approved by the FDA in 2004 for treating lipoatrophy resulting from medications used in HIV-positive patients [37]. Since then it has been used off-label to revolumize the skin in cosmetic patients. PLLA is one of several fillers currently available that stimulate fibroblasts to produce collagen. An-other is ArteFill (Artes Medical, San Diego, CA), which is still awaiting FDA approval. This agent is composed of microscopic spheres of polyme-thylmethacrylate (PMMA) mixed with purified bovine collagen [38]. It is in-jected under the skin, where it remains permanently to encourage the formation of collagen. Over time, the bovine collagen portion is absorbed, whereas the microspheres remain. These collagen stimulating fillers are both used to treat deep nasolabial folds.

The latest filler to be approved by the FDA is an injectable compound of calcium hydroxylapatite microspheres suspended in an aqueous carboxy-methylcellulose gel. Each of these components has been used in implants and drug delivery systems for many years; the current indications evolved from experience with use in dentistry, orthopedics, urology, and neurosurgery [39]. Marketed as Radiesse (BioForm Medical, Inc., San Mateo, CA), it is ap-proved for treating moderate to severe facial rhytids, such as in the nasolabial folds. Once injected, the vehicle slowly starts to degrade and collagen deposi-tion begins to occur around the microspheres, resulting in tissue expansion and a consistency similar to that of the surrounding tissue. Over time, the mi-crospheres become part of the adjacent soft tissue and are anchored in place, allowing for longevity, with correction durations of up to a year or more [40].

Although not a filler, botulinum toxin-A, or Botox (Allergan, Inc., Irvine, CA), is a naturally occurring exotoxin produced by *Clostridium botulinum*, which prevents local neuromuscular transmission. When injected into glabel-lar folds, it inhibits muscle contraction. Although botulinum toxin does not directly reverse changes from photodamage, it gives the appearance of rejuve-nation by relaxing the underlying musculature. In a large placebo-controlled trial, it was shown to significantly reduce the severity of glabellar lines [41].

Finally, some of the earliest fillers involved the use of collagen itself. First used in the 1980s, the early collagen fillers were derived from bovine sources. Zyplast (Allergan, Inc., Irvine, CA) and Cosmoderm/Cosmoplast (Inamed Corporation, Santa Barbara, CA) require skin testing for potential hyper-sensitivity weeks before the injection, and results last only a few months [42]. The FDA is currently considering the application of a new collagen filler, Evolence (Canderm, Montreal, Quebec, Canada), which is derived from pork tendons. Available in Canada, Europe, and elsewhere, this product is attractive because it is nonallergic and compatible with human collagen, and therefore will not require preprocedure skin testing [43].

Chemical peels

Chemical peels are classified as superficial, medium, and deep according to the depth or penetration, the agent used, and the time it remains on the skin [44]. Superficial peels are usually performed with glycolic acid in concentrations between 40% and 70%, which penetrates the epidermis. Usually three to five treatments are required for optimal results. However, part of its popularity is the ability of most patients to return to work the same day, hence the nickname *lunchtime peel*. Trichloroacetic acid (TCA) is considered a medium-depth peeling agent, because it penetrates through the epidermis and into the upper dermis. It is prescribed for deeper wrinkles and more severe damage, and patients may require up to a week before resuming work.

Deep peels are usually performed with phenol, a chemical used for this purpose since the nineteenth century. Phenol produces dramatic results because it penetrates deep into the dermis. However, it is toxic to the kidneys, liver, and heart, and therefore candidates for a phenol peel must be carefully evaluated (Table 2).

Microdermabrasion

Microdermabrasion is another option to treat photoaged skin. It involves the use of sprays of fine crystal particles to abrade the skin through a closed loop system that contains a vacuum to aspirate used particles and skin debris. The depth of abrasion depends on the type of crystals used, the number of passes the operator makes along the treated area, and the type of machine. Approximately 838,000 cases of microdermabrasion were performed in the United States in 2005 [45]. This superficial cosmetic procedure has been shown to temporarily improve many skin problems,

Table 2
Commonly used chemical peels

Type of peel	Agent used	Indications	Recovery time
Superficial	Glycolic acid	Fine wrinkles Irregular pigmentation Rough texture	1–3 days
Medium	Trichloroacetic acid	Remove precancerous lesions Irregular pigmentation	7–10 days
Deep	Phenol	Deep wrinkles Remove precancerous lesions	Several weeks

including mottled pigmentation, fine wrinkles, and skin texture irregularities. In addition, recent studies have shown that the abrasive component of microdermabrasion stimulates the expression of key genes involved in dermal remodeling, which may be key in achieving and retaining the desired results [46].

Laser systems

Finally, laser resurfacing is used to reduce fine wrinkles and other minor imperfections, especially around the mouth and eyes. The laser beam vaporizes damaged cells by emitting bursts of radiation or heat energy that are absorbed by water in the cells. Many applications for cutaneous laser surgery exist for treating aging and photoaged skin. These conditions include the treatment of telangiectasia, hyperpigmentation, and dermal remodeling. Both ablative and nonablative lasers have been used successfully to treat photoaging, partially to help increase collagen production [47].

Ablative systems include the carbon dioxide (CO_2) and erbium/yttrium aluminum-garnet (YAG) lasers. Facial resurfacing with the CO_2 laser is considered the gold standard and typically produces at least a 50% improvement in skin tone, wrinkle severity, and scar depth. The more recently developed erbium/YAG laser has shown comparable results with fewer side effects than the CO_2 laser [48]. These ablative systems have the potential to cause hypertrophic scar formation and pigmentary changes. Down time can last at least a week, with full recovery occurring a month or more postprocedure.

Nonablative laser systems work to encourage collagen production and dermal remodeling by creating a dermal wound without disruption of the epidermis. They are less effective than ablative systems when treating photoaging but can reduce hyperpigmentation and telangiectasia. Intense pulsed light (IPL) is a popular nonablative system. Although not classified as lasers, IPL systems target pigmentation in the epidermis, such as that found in solar lentigines and telangiectasia, to achieve a younger and fresher appearance of the skin [49]. One of the newest nonablative lasers is the fractional resurfacing laser, or Fraxel (Reliant Technologies, Inc., Mountain View, CA). Unlike conventional lasers, this technology produces superheated microscopic columns of thermal damage or microthermal zones (MTZs) in the dermis. It is approved by the FDA for treating rhytids, melasma, surgical and acne scars, skin resurfacing, and striae. Its target, or chromophore, is water, and therefore it penetrates the stratum corneum and into the dermis to create a wound-healing response and remodeling of collagen [50].

Another popular means of treating the laxity that results from aging and photoaging is radio frequency technology. These devices produce an electric current that generates heat through resistance in the dermis and subcutaneous tissue. Clinical changes are believed to result from collagen contraction, which is followed by secondary collagen synthesis and dermal remodeling

[51]. Thermage (Thermage, Inc., Hayward, CA) is one of the most popular devices used for this treatment.

Sunscreens

Aging skin results from intrinsic, or nonpreventable, factors and extrinsic, or preventable, causes. The extrinsic cause most easily prevented is exposure to sunlight. Sun exposure harms the skin through the effects of UV radiation; UVB causes redness of the skin, whereas UVA penetrates deeper into the dermis and causes more DNA damage. This exposure results in a significant effect on collagen production and pigmentation and is responsible for skin thickening, mottled pigmentation, and wrinkling. Although some exposure is unavoidable, avoiding the sun between 10 AM and 3 PM, using physical barriers such as hats and clothing, and using sunscreen regularly are recommended to minimize photoaging and damage [52].

In the United States, sunscreen agents are regulated by the FDA as OTC medications and protect the skin by absorbing, scattering, or reflecting UVA and UVB rays. The current FDA sunscreen monograph, issued in 1999, includes 16 agents [53]. Fourteen of these agents are organic absorbers/filters, which is the recommended terminology for what were formerly called *chemical* filters. The remaining two agents are titanium dioxide and zinc oxide, which physically block UV rays from penetrating the skin and are now referred to as *inorganic absorbers/fillers*. Although sunscreens are now included in many cosmetics, such as moisturizers and foundations, it is important to ensure the sunscreen used is appropriate for the type of skin to be protected.

The FDA requires that all sunscreens contain a label indicating the sun protection factor (SPF). Used in the United States since 1978, SPF indicates the relative amount of protection against sunburn that a sunscreen can provide when used properly by the average user. SPF is determined by dividing the time of UVB exposure needed to produce erythema with sunscreen by the time of UVB exposure needed to produce erythema on unprotected skin. For example, if an individual normally burns in 20 minutes, SPF 10 would allow 200 minutes of sun exposure before burning the skin. Thus, the shorter time needed to produce erythema, the higher the SPF required. Most experts recommend using at least an SPF 15. Although some people believe that two applications of SPF 15 provides twice the protection, or SPF 30, compared to a single application of SPF 15, that is not the case. In order to achieve an SPF of 30, an individual must use a product labeled as such.

Furthermore, the current 1999 FDA monograph sets standards for labeling sunscreens according to their resistance to water immersion. To be labeled as *water resistant*, a sunscreen must maintain its SPF after 40 minutes of water immersion, whereas *very water resistant* sunscreens must maintain their SPF after 80 minutes in the water.

Although SPF ratings apply to the UVB wavelength, no universally accepted rating system exists for UVA protection [54]. Until recently, sunscreen labeled *broad spectrum* and containing avobenzone or oxybenzone was recommended to provide the most chemical protection from UVA rays. Two new agents were recently approved by the FDA. The first, Helioplex, is a combination of avobenzone, oxybenzone, and a photostabilizing agent. It can be found in several Neutrogena products. The second is Mexoryl, marketed in the United States as Anthelios SX (LaRoche-Posay, Morristown, NJ), which has been popular in Europe for many years but was not approved by the FDA until 2006. One advantage of these new compounds is their stability in the presence of UVA radiation compared with older UVA sunscreens.

The newest class of sunscreens combines the benefits of inorganic and organic filters. Agents in this class absorb UV radiation similar to organic compounds (the former *chemical blockers*) and also scatter and reflect rays like inorganic agents (formerly referred to as *physical blockers*). Although available in Europe and elsewhere, the FDA has not approved sunscreens in this class for United States consumers [55].

For UV protection to be effective, certain guidelines should be followed. First, because it must be absorbed into the skin to be effective, sunscreen should be applied at least 20 minutes before sun exposure and must be reapplied at regular intervals if exposure is prolonged. It should be applied liberally and evenly to provide maximum coverage. Lipsticks and other lip preparations should also contain sunscreen. A good sunscreen for sensitive skin is one that does not use chemicals but rather contains titanium dioxide or zinc oxide, which physically blocks UV radiation like a piece of clothing.

Finally, although the current emphasis is on avoiding ultraviolet radiation, many consumers still feel more comfortable about their appearance when it includes a "tanned look." Manufacturers have responded to this with oral and topical products designed to produce an artificial tan. Tanning pills, such as those found in health food stores, are not approved by the FDA and have side effects ranging from nausea and diarrhea to drug-induced hepatitis. At least one death was reported from aplastic anemia in a woman using tanning pills [56]. Sunless tanners, however, are safe to use. The only color additive currently approved by the FDA for sunless tanning is dihydroxyacetone (DHA), which works by reacting with amino acids in the skin to produce a temporary, artificial tan [57]. The amount of color an individual develops depends on several factors, including the number of times it is applied, the shade chosen, and body chemistry. In addition, to achieve optimal results, proper preparation of the skin is recommended, including exfoliating the skin to be tanned, such as with an alpha hydroxy acid or washcloth; applying the product to clean, dry skin; and washing the hands with soap and water immediately after application. However, although users may look as if they spent a day at the beach, neither self-tanning preparations nor the artificial tan produced protects the skin from UV injury. Although DHA offers some protection against UVA through its oxidation effect that changes skin color to tan, tanning induced by DHA results only in an SPF of 2. Therefore, sunscreen must be used in the presence of a "DHA tan."

In summary, not all the visible signs associated with aging are inevitable, nor must they be a permanent part of one's appearance. Avoiding sunlight and other environmental toxins remains the single most important factor to prevent an aged appearance. A wide variety of products and treatments are currently available to treat these skin changes, with more being developed as consumers recognize that chronologic age does not always have to show on their skin.

References

[1] Yaar M, Gilchrest BA. Aging of skin. In: Freedberg IM, Eisen AZ, Wolff K, et al, editors. Fitzpatrick's dermatology in general medicine. New York: McGraw-Hill; 2003. p. 1386–98.
[2] Stiller MJ, Bartolone J, Stern R, et al. Topical 8% glycolic acid and 8% L-Lactic acid creams for the treatment of photodamaged skin. Arch Dermatol 1996;132:631–6.
[3] Lavker RM. Cutaneous aging: chronologic versus photoaging. In: Gilchrest BA, editor. Photodamage. Cambridge (UK): Blackwell Science; 1995. p. 123–35.
[4] Elson ML. Use of tretinoin in female health practice. Int J Fertil 1998;43(2):117–21.
[5] Quan T, He T, Shao Y, et al. Elevated cysteine-rich 61 mediates aberrant collagen homeostasis in chronologically aged and photoaged human skin. Am J Pathol 2006;169(2):482–90.
[6] Kligman D. Cosmeceuticals. Dermatol Clin 2000;18:609–15.
[7] Brody HJ. Relevance of cosmeceuticals to the dermatologic surgeon. Dermatol Surg 2005; 31:796–8.
[8] Clark CP III. Alpha hydroxy acids in skin care. Clin Plast Surg 1996;23:49–56.
[9] Kneedler JA, Sky SS, Sexton LR. Understanding alpha-hydroxy acids. Dermatol Nurs 1998; 10(4):247–62.
[10] Roth AC. Benefits of AHAs stem from an increase in dermal perfusion. Cosmetic Dermatology 1996;10(Suppl):11.
[11] Ditre CM. Exfoliants: AHAs and BHAs. In: Draelos ZD, editor. Cosmeceuticals. 1st edition. Philadelphia: Saunders; 2005. p. 111–8.
[12] Bernstain EF, Brown DB, Schwartz MD, et al. The polyhydroxy acid gluconolactone protects against ultraviolet radiation in an in vitro model of cutaneous photoaging. Dermatol Surg 2004;30:189–96.
[13] Kang S, Duell EA, Fisher GJ, et al. Application of retinol to human skin in vivo induces epidermal hyperplasia and cellular retinoid binding proteins characteristic of retinoic acid but without measurable retinoic acid levels or irritation. J Invest Dermatol 1995;105(4):549–56.
[14] Glaser DA. Anti-aging products and cosmeceuticals. Facial Plast Surg Clin North Am 2003; 11:219–27.
[15] Kang S, Fisher GJ, Voorhees JJ. Photoaging and topical tretinoin: therapy, pathogenesis, and prevention. Arch Dermatol 1997;133(10):1280–4.
[16] Humbert PG, Haftek M, Creidi P, et al. Topical ascorbic acid on photoaged skin. Clinical, topographical and ultrastructural evaluation: double blind study vs. placebo. Exp Dermatol 2003;12:237–44.
[17] Lin FH, Lin JY, Gupta RD, et al. Ferulic acid stabilizes a solution of vitamins c and e and doubles its photoprotection of skin. J Invest Dermatol 2005;125:826–32.
[18] Beitner H. Randomized, placebo-controlled, double blind study on the clinical efficacy of a cream containing 5% alpha lipoic acid related to photoaging of facial skin. Br J Dermatol 2003;68:841–9.

[19] Shindo Y, Witt E, Han D, et al. Enzymic and non-enzymic antioxidants in epidermis and dermis of human skin. J Invest Dermatol 1994;102:122–4.

[20] Imada I, Fujita T, Sugiyama Y, et al. Effects of idebenone and related compounds on respiratory activities of brain mitochrondria, and on lipid peroxidation of their membranes. Arch Gerontol Geriatr 1989;8:323–41.

[21] Rattan SI, Clark BF. Kinetin delays the onset of aging characteristics in human fibroblasts. Biochem Biophys Res Commun 1994;201:665–72.

[22] Katiyar SK, Ahmad N, Mukhtar H. Green tea and skin. Arch Dermatol 2000;136:989–94.

[23] McDaniel DH, Neudecker BA, Dinardo JC, et al. Idebenone: a new antioxidant–Part I. Relative assessment of oxidative stress protection capacity compared to commonly known antioxidants. J Cosmet Dermatol 2005;4(1):10–7.

[24] Harding KG, Moore K, Phillips TJ. Wound chronicity and fibroblast senescence: implications for treatment. Int Wound J 2005;2(4):364–8.

[25] Ignotz RA, Endo T, Massague J. Regulation of fibronectin and type I collagen mRNA levels by transforming growth factor-beta. J Biol Chem 1987;262(14):6443–6.

[26] Mustoe TA, Pierce GF, Thomason A, et al. Accelerated healing of incisional wounds in rats induced by transforming growth factor-beta. Science 1987;237(4820):1333–6.

[27] Katayama K, Armendariz-Borunda J, Raghow R, et al. A pentapeptide from type I procollagen promotes extracellular matrix production. J Biol Chem 1993;268(14):9941–4.

[28] Dahiya A, Romano JF. Cosmeceuticals: a review of their use for aging and photoaged skin. Cosmetic Dermatology 2006;19(7):479–84.

[29] Grimes PE. Melasma. Etiologic and therapeutic considerations. Arch Dermatol 1995;131(12):1453–7.

[30] Rendon M, Berneburg M, Arellano I, et al. Treatment of melasma. J Am Acad Dermatol 2006;54(5 Suppl 2):S272–81.

[31] Garcia A, Fulton JE. The combination of glycolic acid and hydroquinone or kojic acid for the treatment of melasma and related conditions. Dermatol Surg 1996;22:443–7.

[32] Sudel KM, Venzke K, Mielke H, et al. Novel aspects of intrinsic and extrinsic aging of human skin: beneficial effects of soy extract. Photochem Photobiol 2005;81(3):581–7.

[33] Brown MB, Jones SA. Hyaluronic acid: a unique topical vehicle for the localized delivery of drugs to the skin. J Eur Acad Dermatol Venereol 2005;19(3):308–18.

[34] Weindl G, Schaller M, Schafer-Korting M, et al. Hyaluronic acid in the treatment and prevention of skin diseases: molecular biological, pharmaceutical and clinical aspects. Skin Pharmacol Physiol 2004;17(5):207–13.

[35] Duranti F, Salti G, Bovani B, et al. Injectable hyaluronic acid gel for soft tissue augmentation: a clinical and histological study. Dermatol Surg 1998;24:1317–25.

[36] Carruthers J, Carruthers A. Hyaluronic acid gel in skin rejuvenation. J Drugs Dermatol 2006;5(10):959–63.

[37] Available at: http://www.sculptra.com/US/resources/pr_20040803.pdf. Accessed July 15, 2007.

[38] Lemperle G, Romano JJ, Busso M. Soft tissue augmentation with artecoll: 10 year history, indications, techniques and complications. Dermatol Surg 2003;29:573–87.

[39] Hubbard W. Bioform implants: biocompatibility. Franksville (WI): BioForm Medical Inc; 2003.

[40] Feldermann LI. Radiesse® for facial rejuvenation. Cosmetic Dermatology 2005;18(12):1–4.

[41] Carruthers JA, Lowe NJ, Menter MA, et al. A multicenter, double blind, randomized, placebo-controlled study of the efficacy and safety of botulinum toxin type A in the treatment of glabellar lines. J Am Acad Dermatol 2002;46:840–9.

[42] Stegman SJ, Chu S, Armstrong R. Adverse reactions to bovine collagen implant: clinical and histologic features. J Dermatol Surg Oncol 1988;14:39–48.

[43] Available at: http://www.evolence.com/prof_how_works.asp. Accessed July 15, 2007.

[44] Burris LM, Roenigk HH Jr. Chemical peel as a treatment for skin damage from excessive sun exposure. Dermatol Nurs 1997;9(2):99–104.

[45] Available at: http://www.plasticsurgery.org/media/statistics/loader.cfm?url=/commonspot/security/getfile.cfm&PageID=17888. Accessed December 30, 2006.

[46] Karimipour DJ, Kang S, Johnson TM, et al. Microdermabrasion with and without aluminum oxide crystal abrasion: a comparative molecular analysis of dermal remodeling. J Am Acad Dermatol 2006;54:405–10.

[47] Tanzi EL, Lupton JR, Alster TS. Lasers in dermatology: four decades of progress. J Am Acad Dermatol 2003;49:1–31.

[48] Tanzi EL, Alster TS. Single pass carbon dioxide versus multiple-pass Er:YAG laser skin resurfacing: a comparison of postoperative wound healing and side-effect rates. Dermatol Surg 2003;29(1):80–4.

[49] Fodor L, Peled IJ, Rissin Y, et al. Using intense pulsed light for cosmetic purposes: our experience. Plast Reconstr Surg 2004;113(6):1789–95.

[50] Manstein D, Herron GS, Sink RK, et al. Fractional photothermolysis: a new concept for cutaneous remodeling using microscopic patterns of thermal injury. Lasers Surg Med 2004;34(5):426–38.

[51] Zellickson BD, Kist D, Bernstein E, et al. Histological and ultrastructural evaluation of the effects of a radiofrequency-based nonablative dermal remodeling device: a pilot study. Arch Dermatol 2004;140:204–9.

[52] Hill L, Ferrini RL. Skin cancer prevention and screening: summary of the American college of preventive medicine's practice policy statements. CA Cancer J Clin 1998;48(4):232–5.

[53] Federal Register: rules and regulations. Fed Regist 1999;64(98):27687–90.

[54] Lim HW, Naylor M, Honigsmann H, et al. American Academy of Dermatology consensus conference on UVA protection of sunscreens: summary and recommendations. Washington DC; Feb 4, 2000. J Am Acad Dermatol 2001;44:505–8.

[55] Reisch MS. New-wave sunscreens. Chem Eng News 2005;83(15):18–22.

[56] Fitzpatrick JE, Aeling JL. Dermatology secrets. Philadelphia: Hanley and Belfus; 1996. p. 315–9.

[57] Johnson JA, Fusaro RM. Broad-spectrum photoprotection: the roles of tinted auto windows, sunscreens and browning agents in the diagnosis and treatment of photosensitivity. Dermatology 1992;185:237–41.

ELSEVIER
SAUNDERS

Nurs Clin N Am 42 (2007) 501–506

NURSING
CLINICS
OF NORTH AMERICA

Index

Note: Page numbers of article titles are in **boldface** type.

Moving?

Make sure your subscription moves with you!

To notify us of your new address, find your **Clinics Account Number** (located on your mailing label above your name), and contact customer service at:

E-mail: elspcs@elsevier.com

800-654-2452 (subscribers in the U.S. & Canada)
407-345-4000 (subscribers outside of the U.S. & Canada)

Fax number: 407-363-9661

Elsevier Periodicals Customer Service
6277 Sea Harbor Drive
Orlando, FL 32887-4800

*To ensure uninterrupted delivery of your subscription, please notify us at least 4 weeks in advance of move.